TECHNICAL REPORT

Building Partner Health Capacity with U.S. Military Forces

Enhancing AFSOC Health Engagement Missions

David E. Thaler • Gary Cecchine • Anny Wong • Timothy Jackson

Prepared for the United States Air Force
Approved for public release; distribution unlimited

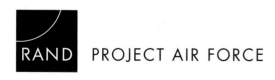

RAND PROJECT AIR FORCE

The research described in this report was sponsored by the United States Air Force under Contract FA7014-06-C-0001. Further information may be obtained from the Strategic Planning Division, Directorate of Plans, Hq USAF.

Library of Congress Cataloging-in-Publication Data

Building partner health capacity with U.S. military forces : enhancing AFSOC health engagement missions / David E. Thaler ... [et al.].
   p. cm.
 Includes bibliographical references.
 ISBN 978-0-8330-6846-0 (pbk. : alk. paper)
 1. United States. Air Force—Medical care. 2. Medicine, Military—United States. 3. Missions, Medical.
4. Technical assistance, American. I. Thaler, David E.

UG983.B85 2012
362.1—dc23

2012026080

Published 2012 by the RAND Corporation
1776 Main Street, P.O. Box 2138, Santa Monica, CA 90407-2138
1200 South Hayes Street, Arlington, VA 22202-5050
4570 Fifth Avenue, Suite 600, Pittsburgh, PA 15213-2665
RAND URL: http://www.rand.org/
To order RAND documents or to obtain additional information, contact
Distribution Services: Telephone: (310) 451-7002;
Fax: (310) 451-6915; Email: order@rand.org

Preface

In 2009, the U.S. Air Force Special Operations Command (AFSOC) unveiled a new concept for a systematic approach to building health capacity in partner countries of strategic importance to the United States. The central premise of the concept is that rather than using U.S. military medical presence in developing countries to directly treat indigenous communities and supplement or replace inadequate local care, U.S. advisors would engage and train local health workers in a systematic and sustained way through health-focused security cooperation. The objectives of these efforts would be to improve the ability of local governments to deliver services, to obviate the need for outside assistance, to enhance the legitimacy of local authorities and providers in the eyes of their citizens, and to prevent the establishment of extremist groups that seek to exploit the absence of government services. The AFSOC concept acknowledges that the U.S. military, in association with other organizations, has a role in helping to improve health care in vulnerable communities in order to improve the security of those communities.

In fall 2009, the AFSOC Surgeon General's office asked RAND to assist in the implementation of its concept. This report reviews Department of Defense guidance and the experience of other organizations and introduces a framework to help AFSOC and the theater commands it supports to plan for, assess, and enhance the effectiveness of building partner capacity in health to improve public health and the provision of health services. These efforts, in turn, can support the extension of good governance and efforts to counter insurgent and terrorist infiltration, recruitment, and exploitation of vulnerable populations.

This report should be of interest to planners in combatant and component commands, the U.S. military medical community, and other U.S. military organizations involved in security cooperation and building the capacity of partner nations.

RAND Project AIR FORCE

RAND Project AIR FORCE (PAF), a division of the RAND Corporation, is the U.S. Air Force's federally funded research and development center for studies and analyses. PAF provides the Air Force with independent analyses of policy alternatives affecting the development, employment, combat readiness, and support of current and future air, space, and cyber forces. Research is conducted in four programs: Force Modernization and Employment; Manpower, Personnel, and Training; Resource Management; and Strategy and Doctrine.

Additional information about PAF is available on our website:
http://www.rand.org/paf/

Contents

Figure and Tables

Figure

Tables

Summary

The U.S. Department of Defense (DoD) has emphasized that strengthening the will, legitimacy, and capabilities of partner governments and security forces and operating "by, with, and through" them are critical to combating insurgent and terrorist groups around the world. A central element of these efforts is influencing "relevant populations" by supporting the extension of governance, rule of law, and basic services to areas that are undergoverned and vulnerable to exploitation by extremist organizations. Health security is part and parcel of a community's overall well-being, and improving it can help enhance government legitimacy while making extremist groups less attractive to citizens.

The study reported here was undertaken to assist the U.S. Air Force Special Operations Command (AFSOC) in executing its recently developed approach to planning for, assessing, and enhancing the effectiveness of missions for building partner capacity in health (BPC-H). BPC-H is defined herein as systematic, long-term missions to enhance the ability of governments to deliver essential medical, dental, and veterinary services to vulnerable populations in developing states that are important to U.S. interests. The premise of this approach is that helping to improve local public health and the provision of health services supports the extension of good governance and counters insurgent and terrorist infiltration, recruitment, and exploitation. AFSOC believes that its health assets can be more effectively and systematically used by combatant commanders in achieving their theater security cooperation objectives, in conjunction with other organizations, such as the U.S. Agency for International Development (USAID). From a broad U.S. government perspective, BPC-H is intended to be used as a stepping-stone to building strong partnerships with individuals and nations that are important to achieving U.S. national security objectives.

This report documents the results of three research tasks:

- place health security in the context of U.S. strategy and security cooperation efforts
- draw lessons from outside organizations on ways U.S. military forces can maximize their effectiveness in helping build partner health capacity
- offer a framework for planning and executing BPC-H missions based on these lessons.

The Gap Between BPC-H Guidance and Practice

There is ample guidance and direction from DoD on the military's role in building partner health capacity to deliver essential medical, dental, and veterinary services to populations in need. Recent DoD guidance clearly directs the military "to be prepared to perform any tasks assigned to establish, reconstitute, and maintain health sector capacity and capability for the indigenous population when indigenous, foreign, or U.S. civilian professionals cannot do so" (U.S. Department of Defense, 2010d, p. 2). Analysis suggests that such services play a critical role in good governance, development, *and* security.[1]

However, despite the importance DoD guidance places on health security and on building partner health capacity, few military medical operations are planned and executed to help accomplish this task and sustain local capacity, except in Iraq and Afghanistan. U.S. military organizations regularly conduct medical missions worldwide, but the vast majority of these missions provide direct delivery of health care to indigenous populations. In some operations, such as disaster response and joint training exercises, efforts are understandably constrained by budgets, legal authorities, the focus on the immediate needs of the population, and the operational requirements of the military mission at hand. However, other missions, including medical civic action programs (MEDCAPs) designed to gain and maintain access to strategically important areas, are often misinterpreted as successful capacity building.

Experiences of Other Organizations

RAND reviewed the relevant experiences of a limited number of outside organizations to provide observations and insights applicable to AFSOC's approach to BPC-H. These organizations included the 95th Civil Affairs Brigade (95th CA BDE), AFSOC's 6th Special Operations Squadron (6th SOS), and Project HOPE (Health Opportunities for People Everywhere), a nongovernmental organization (NGO). The 95th CA BDE was selected because it is a Special Operations organization that conducts health activities in austere environments and contributes to DoD's partnership-building efforts through civil-military engagement (CME) missions. The 6th SOS was selected because of its relatively long history in building partner aviation capacity in less-developed nations. Project HOPE has operated in more than 100 countries to strengthen health infrastructure, train medical professionals, and provide humanitarian assistance. RAND also consulted with military health experts in DoD, development experts in NGOs, and other professionals to provide as broad a review as possible. These experts offered a number of insights on identifying strategies, selecting techniques, developing programs, and tracking progress relevant to AFSOC's BPC-H approach; these insights inform the findings and recommendations of this study.

A Framework for Planning and Executing BPC-H Missions

AFSOC's pursuit of BPC-H occurs within a political and institutional context that is defined by national and theater security cooperation priorities and objectives. Appropriate metrics can help inform AFSOC's internal planning, resourcing, coordination, monitoring, and evaluation needs. They can also help communicate progress and achievements to external audiences, such as the Pentagon, other federal agencies, governmental and nongovernmental entities in partner nations, local communities in partner nations that stand to benefit from the provision of better

---

[1]   See, for example, Jones et al., 2006, p. xxi.

health services, and organizations active in international health and economic development with whom AFSOC and theater commands might associate.

This study proposes a four-phased conceptual approach to planning for, implementing, and assessing the effectiveness of activities to build partner health capacity:

1. consult, plan, and prepare for start-up
2. launch activities
3. conduct full-scale implementation
4. draw down, transition, and (possibly) withdraw.

Although theater BPC-H activities would generally involve multiyear efforts in specific health sectors (e.g., maternal health) within individual partner nations, this approach could also be applied to regional efforts. In all four phases, input, process, output, and outcome metrics would help planners monitor alignment of implementation with goals and strategy.

Based on direction from the Theater Special Operations Command (TSOC) for Africa (SOCAFRICA), initial BPC-H efforts focus on the African countries that are included in Operation Enduring Freedom–Trans-Sahara (OEF-TS). The efforts involve instructing these nations' military personnel to enable them to provide initial health services to residents in remote regions and possibly help train civilian providers. The framework is described in terms relevant to this mission, and generic metrics are offered for each of the phases. Specific metrics for particular programs would have to be developed on the basis of the goals and progress of those programs.

Key Findings and Recommendations

The study's key findings are summarized below, and a set of recommendations for maximizing the effectiveness of efforts to build partner health capacity is provided. The recommendations are directed to the U.S. Air Force (USAF) in general and to AFSOC and the theater commands it supports in particular.

Key Findings

- **Theater commands are the key to closing the gap between guidance and execution of BPC-H.** The requirement for BPC-H is defined in DoD guidance. Theater commands need to direct BPC-H activities—and source them—in order for guidance to be fulfilled. BPC-H missions are relatively inexpensive, but their return can be substantial in terms of both supporting partners and avoiding the cost of later intervention.
- **Efforts to build partner health capacity can be either *supported* or *supporting* operations.** Depending on the operational context, conditions may exist in some regions or states that preclude the U.S. military from training, advising, and assisting existing or potential partners in "kinetic" (combat) capabilities. BPC-H efforts can help "get a foot in the door" and may be a primary means of gaining access and initiating relationships. DoD Instruction 6000.16 recognizes that the priority of such medical operations is comparable to that of combat operations.

- **The U.S. Air Force can play an important role in building partner military health capacity.** USAF serves as executive agent for the Defense Institute for Medical Operations (DIMO) and provides training in disaster preparedness to foreign countries. Moreover, USAF's International Health Specialists (IHSs), competent not only in medical skills but also in foreign languages and regional knowledge, provide a unique capability for Air Force Major Commands (MAJCOMs) and Geographic Combatant Command (GCC) commanders. Thus, USAF is well-positioned to expand its role in building partner health capacity.
- **AFSOC's BPC-H "niche" in the near term appears to be the mission itself.** Very few military organizations are systematically pursuing BPC-H as defined here, yet the demand is great. While AFSOC advisors may not need to specialize yet, as the broader Air Force meets guidance by organizing, equipping, and training its medical, dental, and veterinary assets to more systematically conduct BPC-H activities, AFSOC advisors will need to define a more specific niche for their capabilities within the mission.
- **Successfully building and sustaining partner health capacity in less-developed regions requires long-term effort and commitment, in synchronization with other military and civilian agencies and organizations, and this may conflict with shorter-term theater command priorities.** Without long-term, focused support for the mission from DoD and the theater commands, BPC-H will be sporadic and may not make the impact that it potentially could make. Sporadic missions may even be counterproductive if they raise expectations that the United States cannot meet.
- **Given the finding immediately above and the need to involve multiple stakeholders in BPC-H efforts, well-defined, multiyear plans are critical to success.** From the outset, plans for enhancing a partner's capacity in a specific health sector must be realistic and based on careful, in-depth assessment of the extant environment in which a BPC-H effort will take place.

Recommendations for AFSOC and USAF

- **Communicate the BPC-H concept and approach repeatedly to external audiences.** AFSOC health advisors will have to communicate the AFSOC concept to generate greater appreciation among key USAF, DoD, and U.S. government stakeholders of the contribution BPC-H can make to both U.S. and partner interests and to establish a consistent resource stream for the mission.
- **In developing plans with theater commands for individual BPC-H programs, schedule multiple visits to the partner nations each year throughout the duration of U.S. military involvement.** Visits should be driven not only by the needs of the plan but also by the high-value relationships that can be built with partner nations over time. Sporadic, infrequent visits neither build nor sustain capacity, nor do they enable solid relationships to form.
- **Engage stakeholders early in the planning process and in program development and design.** Often, partner military capacity in health will be built in the context of efforts by civilian organizations (such as USAID) to work with partner health ministries and civilian medical communities. Moreover, potential associates, such as NGOs, must be included in initial planning, as they need time to prepare for their participation in an activity.

- **Assess BPC-H activities by both military and developmental measures of effectiveness.** AFSOC and the theater commands will need to show success based on both developmental and military metrics to continue generating support for the BPC-H mission among existing and potential stakeholders.
- **Approach early BPC-H excursions with an eye toward learning lessons and adapting procedures based on experience.** Engagement in OEF-TS countries offers an opportunity for the theater commands and AFSOC to critically examine the approach to BPC-H.
- **Consider the "risk" of success.** Given other critical tasks that AFSOC's medical community must perform, including force health protection and casualty care, AFSOC will need to understand and evaluate the trade-offs it is making between BPC-H and other requirements if demand for BPC-H missions rises.
- **Examine whether and how AFSOC's BPC-H concept and approach are scalable to the general-purpose Air Force.** If USAF decides to embrace the mission in a systematic fashion, it will be necessary to examine AFSOC's approach and to understand how it can be applied on a larger scale.
- **Consider dedicating some USAF and/or other MAJCOM-level resources to forming a cadre of medical personnel with regional focus and expertise in BPC-H planning and execution.** USAF might determine whether a cadre of medical personnel dedicated to BPC-H (potentially including an expanded IHS program) is warranted.

Acknowledgments

We wish to thank the many people who supported the study documented in this report. The study sponsor, then–Brig Gen Bart O. Iddins, former Surgeon General of Air Force Special Operations Command (AFSOC/SG), was extremely generous with his time in sharing his vision and insights on health operations. Lt Col Michael Hartzell (former Chief, Irregular Warfare/Medical Stability Operations Division, AFSOC/SGK) was our point of contact and also offered valuable insights and guidance in numerous discussions and in his review of an earlier draft of the report. We wish to express our appreciation to Paula Thornhill, Director of RAND Project AIR FORCE's Strategy and Doctrine Program, for her encouragement of and comments on our work and for the guidance she provided throughout the study. Many thanks also go to Lt Col John Crowe (current Chief, AFSOC/SGK) for his insights and comments and for arranging discussions with personnel at Special Operations Command for Africa (SOCAFRICA) and U.S. Africa Command (USAFRICOM), and to MSgt Martin Vera (AFSOC/SGK) for his support of our visits to AFSOC.

We are indebted to Warner Anderson (OASD/HA/TMA), Col Mylene Huynh (AFMSA/SGXI), Lt Col Louis Goler (AFMSA/SGXI), James O'Neill (Europe Regional Medical Command), Fred Gerber (COL, USA, Ret., Project HOPE), MAJ Ross Lightsey, Sr. (U.S. Army John F. Kennedy Special Warfare Center and School), LTC Jose Madera (U.S. Army Civil Affairs and Psychological Operations Command), Peter Berman (World Bank Group), Eugene Bonventre (RAND), C. O. Pannenborg (World Bank Group), Gery Ryan (RAND), Barney Singer (Academy for Educational Development), and Dillon Smith (Academy for Educational Development). We also gained great insight from personnel at SOCAFRICA and USAFRICOM.

Many thanks go to RAND colleagues Richard Hoffmann and Marla Haims for their reviews. Their suggestions strengthened the report in significant ways.

Finally, we appreciate the considerable support we received from other members of the RAND staff. We thank colleagues Michael Neumann for reviewing and refining briefings, outlines, and a draft of this report; Judy Siegel for finalizing the draft for dissemination; Francisco Walter for helping prepare the manuscript; and Janet DeLand for editing the final report.

Responsibility for the content of the report lies solely with the authors.

Abbreviations

6th SOS	6th Special Operations Squadron
95th CA BDE	95th Civil Affairs Brigade
AFSOC	Air Force Special Operations Command
AFSOC/SG	Air Force Special Operations Command/Surgeon General
BPC	building partner capacity
BPC-H	building partner capacity in health
CAA	combat aviation advisor
CME	civil-military engagement
CMSE	Civil Military Support Element
COCOM	combatant command
DENTCAP	dental care program
DIMO	Defense Institute for Medical Operations
DoD	Department of Defense
DoDI	Department of Defense Instruction
GCC	Geographic Combatant Command
GPRA	Government Performance and Accountability Act
HA/DR	humanitarian assistance/disaster relief
HOPE	Health Opportunities for People Everywhere
IHS	International Health Specialist
IW	irregular warfare
IW/HE	irregular warfare/health engagement
JCET	Joint/Combined Exchange Training
JTF	Joint Task Force

MAJCOM	Air Force Major Command
MEDCAP	medical civil action program
MEDEVAC	medical evacuation
MEDRETE	medical readiness training exercise
MHS	Military Health System
MSO	medical stability operation
NGO	nongovernmental organization
OAD	operational aviation detachment
OEF	Operation Enduring Freedom
OEF-P	Operation Enduring Freedom–Philippines
OEF-TS	Operation Enduring Freedom–Trans-Sahara
PAF	Project AIR FORCE
SOCAFRICA	Special Operations Command for Africa
SOF	Special Operations Forces
SSTR	stability, security, transition, and reconstruction
TSCTP	Trans-Sahara Counter Terrorism Partnership
TSOC	Theater Special Operations Command
USAF	U.S. Air Force
USAFRICOM	U.S. Africa Command
USAID	U.S. Agency for International Development
USASOC	U.S. Army Special Operations Command
USCENTCOM	U.S. Central Command
USEUCOM	U.S. European Command
USSOCOM	U.S. Special Operations Command
VETCAP	veterinary care program

CHAPTER ONE

Introduction

Former Secretary of Defense Robert M. Gates instructed the U.S. armed forces to prepare to conduct operations against terrorist, insurgent, and other "irregular" threats to U.S. interests around the world for many years to come.[1] As part of this direction, the Department of Defense (DoD) has emphasized that strengthening the will, legitimacy, and capabilities of partner governments and security forces and operating "by, with, and through" them are critical to combating these threats.[2] The most recent defense guidance calls for "working with allies and partners to establish control over ungoverned territories" and using "non-military means and military-to-military cooperation to address instability and reduce the demand for significant U.S. force commitments to stability operations."[3] A central element of these efforts is influencing "relevant populations" by helping local authorities extend governance, rule of law, and basic services to areas that are undergoverned and vulnerable to exploitation by extremist organizations. Thus, the U.S. military must prepare not only to conduct direct action against terrorist and insurgent groups but also to support improvements in the environments in which those populations exist. In a recent *Foreign Affairs* article, Gates wrote:

> In the decades to come, the most lethal threats to the United States' safety and security—a city poisoned or reduced to rubble by a terrorist attack—are likely to emanate from states that cannot adequately govern themselves or secure their own territory. Dealing with such fractured or failing states is, in many ways, the main security challenge of our time. . . . In these situations, the effectiveness and credibility of the United States will only be as good as the effectiveness, credibility, and sustainability of its local partners. (Gates, 2010, p. 1)

The goal of building partner capacity (BPC) is to enable willing nations to counter insurgent and terrorist threats to their own security and to join the United States and other allies in regional activities as members of coalitions. U.S. efforts to build the capacity of Iraqi and Afghan armed forces are the most visible manifestations of BPC, but in many other parts of the world, BPC activities by U.S. military forces are under way to enlist partners in sustaining pressure on transnational extremist groups while minimizing U.S. involvement in combat operations.

Many U.S. military BPC operations are focused on enhancing the capabilities of a country's military forces to conduct security and combat operations. This is certainly appropri-

---

[1]   Recent guidance directs DoD components to "recognize that IW [irregular warfare] is as strategically important as traditional warfare" (U.S. Department of Defense, 2008a).

[2]   See U.S. Department of Defense, 2010a.

[3]   See U.S. Department of Defense, 2012, pp. 1 and 6.

ate. But in developing countries, where many of the populations that are most vulnerable to terrorist or insurgent groups reside, the capacity to govern and provide essential services—not just "kinetic" (or combat) capacity—is in critical need of support from external sources. While it may be difficult to establish a direct link between poverty and the paucity of basic services (medical, water, sanitation, veterinary, etc.) and the tendency of communities to support extremist groups, there is evidence to suggest that such services play a critical role in good governance, development, *and* security. According to a 2006 RAND report on health capacity and nation-building, "security is significantly impacted by the role health plays in helping to win 'hearts and minds.' . . . inability to win hearts and minds [can] contribute to insurgency, warlordism, and an unstable security environment" (Jones et al., 2006, p. xxi).

"Health security" is part and parcel of a community's overall well-being and can help enhance government legitimacy while making extremist groups less attractive to citizens. Many countries with active or latent jihadist or insurgent challenges are also among the poorest; their populations suffer from nutritional deficiencies and disease and lack preventive medical and dental care. Many of these countries also have agrarian-based economies in which animals serve as the cornerstone of subsistence and income, yet veterinary care is inadequate. Under such conditions and in combination with a lack of security, extremist groups can more easily exploit local populations. Even incremental but sustained improvements in services and governance (as part of a holistic approach to enhancing well-being) can help these populations resist such exploitation and can turn their allegiance toward the local authorities.

The study described in this report was undertaken to assist Air Force Special Operations Command (AFSOC) in executing its concept for planning, assessing, and enhancing the effectiveness of building partner capacity in health (BPC-H).[4] BPC-H is defined herein as systematic, long-term missions to enhance the ability of governments in developing states that are important to U.S. interests to deliver essential medical, dental, and veterinary services to vulnerable populations. Helping to improve local public health and the provision of health services supports extension of good governance and counters insurgent and terrorist infiltration, recruitment, and exploitation. AFSOC believes that its health assets can be more effectively and systematically utilized by combatant commanders in support of their theater security cooperation objectives and in conjunction with other organizations such as the U.S. Agency for International Development (USAID). From a broad U.S. government perspective, BPC-H is intended to be used as a stepping-stone to building strong partnerships with individuals and nations that are important to achieving U.S. national security objectives. The increasing DoD emphasis on influencing "relevant populations," combined with AFSOC's concept, creates an impetus for AFSOC to consider new methods of planning, concepts of operation, tactics, techniques, and procedures that maximize its support of these missions in light of U.S. Air Force (USAF), U.S. Special Operations Command (USSOCOM), and Geographic Combatant Command (GCC) requirements; current best practices; and challenges to and opportunities for AFSOC engagement.

This report documents the results of three research tasks:

- place "health security" in the context of U.S. strategy and security cooperation efforts
- draw lessons from outside organizations on ways U.S. military forces can maximize their effectiveness in helping build partner health capacity

---

[4]   The abbreviation BPC-H was coined at RAND.

- offer a framework for planning and executing BPC-H missions based on these lessons.

AFSOC's Concept for Building Partner Health Capacity

Basic health and medical care—which includes dental and veterinary care—is one of the most important services a government can provide its population and a key indicator of government legitimacy. This is especially true in developing states like those on the African continent in which health care is in very short supply and the social safety net is extremely weak or absent. Lack of access to health services can also destabilize governments and leave open the door for terrorist or insurgent groups to win over the populace in the absence of other aid.[5]

Numerous development efforts to improve health in the developing world are ongoing under the auspices of civilian government agencies, international organizations, and nongovernmental organizations (NGOs). USAID, the United Nations, and nongovernmental development groups are putting substantial resources into improving the health of vulnerable populations in Africa and elsewhere. However, U.S. military forces have a role to play in these nations as well. They can improve the ability of local security forces to administer health services not only within their ranks but also among vulnerable populations in contested regions, and they can help enhance local civilian capabilities in support of agencies such as USAID.

Despite DoD guidance to build partner health capacity, described later, the U.S. military's focus has been on short-term, often direct treatment of indigenous populations rather than capacity building. In 2009, AFSOC unveiled a new command concept for a systematic approach to BPC-H. The central premise is that rather than using U.S. military medical presence in developing countries to directly treat indigenous communities, supplementing or replacing inadequate local care, U.S. advisors should instead engage and train local military and civilian health professionals in a systematic and sustained way. The objectives of these efforts would be to improve the ability of local governments to deliver services, obviating the need for outside assistance; to enhance the legitimacy of local authorities and providers in the eyes of their citizens; and to deny ready access to terrorist and insurgent groups. The AFSOC concept acknowledges that such improvements often take years of sustained effort and that careful planning with and within the theater commands that AFSOC supports—as well as the U.S. Department of State/USAID, the partner governments, and other associated parties—is a prerequisite for the success of both individual BPC-H efforts and for the sustainment of capabilities for such efforts in the U.S. military. In this report, a *partner* is the foreign government that is the target of capacity-building efforts; an *associate* is an agency, organization, or ally that works with AFSOC and the theater command to plan and execute the mission in the partner nation.

AFSOC is already moving forward to initiate its initial BPC-H programs. Working with commanders and planners in U.S. Africa Command (USAFRICOM) and Special Operations Command for Africa (SOCAFRICA), U.S. military health advisors have undertaken programs in the West African countries that are included in Operation Enduring Freedom–Trans-Sahara (OEF-TS).[6] The efforts involve instruction to these nations' military personnel to enable them

---

[5] For more information about how the absence of health care can destabilize nations, see Cecchine and Moore, 2006.

[6] OEF-TS provides military support to the Department of State's Trans-Sahara Counter Terrorism Partnership (TSCTP) program, an integrated, multiyear, multiagency initiative to combat the spread of extremist ideology in the region. The U.S.

to provide initial health services to residents in remote regions and possibly help train civilian providers. OEF-TS aims to strengthen the capabilities of partner nations in the region to control their own territories and to enhance regional cooperation and interoperability, thereby denying al Qaeda affiliates and other violent extremist groups sanctuary in the Sahara and the Sahel. Other programs are under consideration in eastern African nations as well.

One element of AFSOC's approach is having small teams of U.S. health advisors train partner personnel not only on the medical, dental, or veterinary issue at hand but also on instructing other health-care providers. Where appropriate, U.S. advisors may provide equipment and required training on how to operate and maintain that equipment. The aim is to create a cadre of competent partner instructors and provide partner nations with a self-sustaining, enhanced capability in given health sectors.

BPC-H Within Existing Force and Command Structures

In 2009, with the support of the Surgeon General of the Air Force, AFSOC established a new division in its Surgeon General's office to develop and implement an overarching health engagement concept. The division's mission is to plan, coordinate, and de-conflict AFSOC health engagement and medical support for IW and stability operations and to serve as medical stability operation (MSO) subject-matter experts for AFSOC, USSOCOM, and USAF (Iddins, undated, p. 19). The division works through the Theater Special Operations Commands (TSOCs) to execute health-engagement medical planning in support of the GCC's theater-engagement strategy, to improve partner nations' delivery of health services to indigenous populations, and to achieve long-term BPC objectives (AFSOC, 2009b). It is committed to the development of discrete health sectors in specific regions for extended time periods and to maintaining intimate knowledge of the personnel, culture, language, social environment, and health-care systems in those areas.

AFSOC is using organic medical capabilities, drawing from a pool of 750 AFSOC personnel that includes clinical nurses, family physicians, psychologists, dentists, medical materiel technicians, and other medical specialists.[7] To support the goals of BPC-H, AFSOC has developed a dedicated medical training pipeline to "standardize and centrally manage all AFSOC medical training, [conduct] classroom and field training for SOF [Special Operations Forces]–specific medical and tactical combat skills training, [and] ensure [that] AFSOC medics [are] trained for SOF missions, including IW/HE [health engagement]/SSTR [stability, security, transition, and reconstruction] operations" (AFSOC, 2009a, pp. 2–3). A key element of this training is the planning and execution of BPC-H missions in challenging physical and cultural environments and in the context of dissimilar health-care systems.

As a component command of USSOCOM, AFSOC must meet the operational requirements and taskings of the TSOCs, usually in coordination with the GCC in support of its theater-engagement priorities. Thus, to pursue AFSOC's BPC-H concept, AFSOC health advisors must operate through a command construct in which they do not control the type, timing, or locations of the missions to which they are assigned. Advisors must plan and execute

---

OEF-TS partners are Algeria, Burkina Faso, Chad, Mali, Mauritania, Morocco, Niger, Nigeria, Senegal, and Tunisia (U.S. Africa Command, undated).

[7]   When appropriate, AFSOC may request augmentation from medical assets in USAF general-purpose forces.

BPC-H missions under the guidance and direction of theater commands. Successful BPC-H requires long-term planning and commitments to partner nations and other stakeholders, and BPC-H programs must be initiated by a TSOC or GCC. However, the paucity of previous BPC-H efforts suggests that theater commands rarely request such dedicated missions. One challenge to building and sustaining partner health-care capacity is the length of time that building health security takes in developing nations. This requirement may not mesh well with the time horizons and focus of GCCs and TSOCs, which tend by nature and even necessity to focus on immediate operational needs and must constantly balance competing priorities.[8]

AFSOC has developed at least two solutions to this dilemma. First, it has provided a medical planner to work on SOCAFRICA's staff, which gives AFSOC a seat at the planning table for the region where the need for basic services is greatest and where BPC-H could have the most impact. This partnership offers SOCAFRICA an experienced planner who can help implement the TSOC's health-engagement strategy in its area of operations while providing AFSOC with insights into potential BPC-H missions and opportunities to coordinate with other important actors (e.g., other Services, USAID, NGOs). Second, AFSOC may try to capitalize on opportunities for future BPC-H missions while on more traditional missions, such as medical civil action programs (MEDCAPs[9]). AFSOC's personnel will bring the BPC mindset with them on any mission, not only to help teach and train partner personnel but also to establish relationships and trust that may lead to follow-on activities involving capacity building.[10]

Research Approach and Roadmap to This Report

In helping AFSOC plan for and assess the effectiveness of its BPC-H missions and to facilitate the development of this area of operations, the RAND team pursued three tasks. First, the team examined the status of the BPC-H mission as a requirement in DoD guidance and military strategy. Team members conducted a careful review of key U.S. guidance documents, including the *National Defense Strategy*, the *Guidance for the Employment of the Force*, the *Irregular Warfare Joint Operating Concept*, and *Military Health Support for Stability Operations*. In addition, the team accessed peer-reviewed academic literature, mission reports, and other sources and held discussions with medical experts in U.S. defense and other organizations to assess the effectiveness of previous and ongoing military health engagements. Finally, the team held detailed discussions with AFSOC/SG concerning AFSOC's concept for planning and conducting BPC-H missions in support of USSOCOM and GCC objectives. Chapter Two reports on the findings of this task.

Second, the RAND team analyzed organizations that have pursued activities similar to or otherwise relevant to AFSOC's BPC-H concept to gain insights into successful practices that AFSOC might apply to its own efforts. Three organizations were selected, in consultation

---

[8] However, DoD Instruction (DoDI) 6000.16 (discussed later) should encourage greater focus in GCCs and TSOCs on longer-term medical stability operations.

[9] MEDCAPs, along with actions focused on dental and veterinary care programs (DENTCAPs and VETCAPs, respectively), are civil-military operations that use indigenous military forces and civilian entities to support economic and social development and improve the standing of those forces. They are often conducted with U.S. military doctors, nurses, and other personnel. See U.S. Department of Defense, 2010b, p. 297.

[10] Author discussions with officials at Air Force Special Operations Command/Surgeon General (AFSOC/SG), April 2010.

with AFSOC/SG: the U.S. Army Special Operations Command's 95th Civil Affairs Brigade (95th CA BDE), AFSOC's own 6th Special Operations Squadron (6th SOS), and Project HOPE (Health Opportunities for People Everywhere).[11] The team reviewed publicly available information about each organization and held focused discussions with the organizations' representatives to develop relevant criteria and variables for understanding the organizations' operations and internal or external assessments of effectiveness and best practices. In addition, RAND pursued discussions with other experts in military health and international development to provide further insight into best practices. Chapter Three reviews the experiences of these organizations and summarizes observations of other experts to identify best practices that AFSOC and the theater commands it supports might consider as they build partner health capacity.

---

[11] Each of these organizations has characteristics that are important to AFSOC/SG, as discussed in Chapter Three.

CHAPTER TWO

The Importance of Building Partner Health Capacity in U.S. Military Strategy

In the parlance of counterterrorism, counterinsurgency, and stability operations, U.S. military operations abroad related to kinetic activities comprise a mix of direct and indirect efforts. In direct operations, U.S. forces operate overtly or covertly, hunting down and attacking or disrupting terrorist and insurgent groups, to achieve operational objectives set by U.S. commanders. Indirect operations are aimed at improving the effectiveness of partner nations' combat forces and center on efforts to train, equip, advise, and assist, often through intensive, hands-on training missions in-country to help those governments build capacity and legitimacy. Operational objectives are achieved by, with, and through partner forces that benefit from U.S. BPC programs. The weight of effort over time should shift from direct to indirect operations, reducing the U.S. footprint in the countries involved (since a large U.S. military presence can delegitimize local governments) and enabling partners to maintain their own security and govern their populations (U.S. Department of Defense, 2008c).

In the case of U.S. military health activities in foreign nations, direct operations are efforts designed to deliver care to local populations and provide hands-on training and experience to U.S. medical personnel. Humanitarian assistance, disaster relief, and civil action programs are examples of direct health operations, which are usually short-lived, discrete efforts. Indirect health operations are dedicated to building and sustaining the capacity of partners to deliver enduring care to their populations over the long term—health engagement, or BPC-H. Traditionally, direct operations have dominated U.S. military health operations. While direct operations can help achieve important U.S. objectives (such as gaining intelligence about insurgent groups) and may involve local health-care providers, the indirect approach has shown greater utility in providing skills to local providers to help them deliver medical, dental, and veterinary services to their own communities over the longer term.

This chapter reviews the rationale for the indirect approach, as characterized by dedicated health engagement with partners, and explores the role of AFSOC health advisors in pursuing this approach. The review is intended to describe the context of and motivation for BPC-H efforts.

Building Partner Health Capacity Is a Key Element of Counterinsurgency, Counterterrorism, and Stability Operations

Indirect health operations are receiving increasing emphasis in DoD guidance documents, directives, and instructions, which make clear that the U.S. military has a critical role to play in helping authorities in states vulnerable to insurgency, terrorism, and other forms of instability to extend governance to populations susceptible to extremist elements.

DoD Guidance on Building Partner Health Capacity

DoD is increasingly focused on operating by, with, and through willing, capable partners. The objective is to enable those partners to work independently and with the United States to defeat terrorist and insurgent groups such as al Qaeda and other transnational threats. DoD recognizes that defeating such threats requires influencing "relevant populations" (U.S. Department of Defense, 2010a, p. 13). In particular, partners must be helped to extend governance, rule of law, and basic services to undergoverned areas. A key goal of DoD support to partner nations is increasing the legitimacy of local authorities in the eyes of their populations by engaging with local security forces and supporting other U.S. agencies such as USAID in their programs with local civilians (U.S. Department of Defense, 2010a, p. 36). USSOCOM has echoed this approach. In testimony to the Senate Armed Services Committee in March 2009, its commander, Admiral Eric Olson, stated that

> USSOCOM favors a "populace-centric" approach in lieu of a "threat-centric" approach to national security challenges. More specifically, we believe that SOF must focus on the environmental dynamics and root causes that create today's and tomorrow's threats and adversaries. (Olson, 2009, p. 14)

In addition, the 2010 Quadrennial Defense Review stated that "ineffective governance can create areas that terrorists and insurgents can exploit" and that populations become susceptible to extremist ideologies "when governments struggle to provide basic services" (U.S. Department of Defense, 2010a, p. 24).

Experience in Iraq and Afghanistan illustrated to U.S. decisionmakers the need for enduring U.S. support for efforts to address governance in undergoverned areas, the improvement of which will take years or decades. In a 2005 DoD directive, the Undersecretary of Defense for Policy wrote

> Stability operations are a core U.S. military mission that the Department of Defense shall be prepared to conduct and support. . . . The immediate goal often is to provide the local populace with security, restore essential services, and meet humanitarian needs. The long-term goal is to help develop indigenous capacity for securing essential services. (U.S. Department of Defense, 2005, p. 2)

The May 2010 version of the Irregular Warfare Joint Operating Concept defined an approach that "requires balance between defeating the threats and enhancing a local partner's legitimacy and influence over a population by addressing the causes of conflict and building the partner's ability to provide security, good governance and economic development" (U.S. Department of Defense, 2010c, p. 7). DoD guidance for a U.S. military role in helping partners build their capacity for governance is clear.[1]

There is also ample guidance and direction from DoD on the military's role in building partner health capacity to deliver essential medical, dental, and veterinary services. A

---

[1] These efforts are intended to be complementary to and supportive of goals of the Department of State and other U.S. and international agencies.

DoD document that gives direction to the GCCs and the Services on priorities for operations and efforts to build partner capacity states that "the design of peacetime health activities will create a quantifiable positive impact on the civilian public health sector and build capacity of the partner nation to deliver essential health services to its population" (U.S. Department of Defense, 2008b). A DoD functional needs analysis on the military health system in stability operations identified "medical security cooperation," "medical capacity building," and "health sector stabilization and reconstruction" as key operational scenarios supporting DoD Directive 3000.05, which itself stated the requirement to "ensure DOD medical personnel and capabilities are prepared to meet military and civilian health requirements in stability operations" (U.S. Department of Defense, 2009, p. 13).

Finally, DoDI 6000.16 is the newest and most specific mandate directing the DoD Military Health System (MHS) to organize, train, and equip forces for health engagement and MSOs. It directs DoD to "be prepared to perform any tasks assigned to establish, reconstitute, and maintain health sector capacity and capability for the indigenous population," including "health sector capacity building" (U.S. Department of Defense, 2010d, pp. 2–3). Notably, the instruction also directs the commanders of the GCCs to "incorporate MSOs into campaign plans; theater security cooperation plans; military training, exercises, and planning, including intelligence campaign plans; and intelligence support plans" (U.S. Department of Defense, 2010d, p. 5). Thus, DoD guidance firmly establishes health engagement as a core mission of the MHS.

BPC-H Engagements as Supported Operations

DoDI 6000.16 clearly states that medical stability operations "shall be given priority comparable to combat operations" (U.S. Department of Defense, 2010d, p. 1). As a consequence, depending on the operational requirements of the GCC in a particular environment, efforts to build partner health capacity can be *supported* rather than *supporting* operations. This would occur when the primary task a theater commander assigns to a commander on the ground—such as an officer from the military health service—is focused on enhancing partner health capacity. Supporting commanders, if any, would aid, protect, complement, or sustain the supported commander's force.[2] In other words, the focus of some operations would be on generating quantifiable improvements in health sectors for the sake of enhancing government legitimacy and the long-term well-being of the population. This is distinct from those health activities intended to support other U.S. military operations—for example, by establishing popular acceptance of U.S. military presence or generating voluntary information on insurgent activities from local citizens, or by denying insurgent or terrorist groups the opportunity to curry favor by providing similar services.

In some regions or countries, conditions may preclude the U.S. military from training, advising, and assisting existing or potential partners in kinetic capabilities. Such conditions include wariness of foreign combat troops or advisors due to historical precedent. Health engagement could be a primary means of gaining access to such regions in a nonthreatening way—to "get a foot in the door" and keep it open. Health engagement could also help increase U.S. influence where U.S. forces had been previously unwelcome or where building other partner military capacities is not warranted or is perceived negatively by local populations. In such

---

[2] Adapted from U.S. Department of Defense, 2010b.

cases, rather than facilitating the presence of U.S. troops, building health capacity is the main purpose of an operation (and a supported activity) whose benefit is to *preclude* a later need for U.S. combat troops. The U.S. motivation for helping bring about these improvements is that the cost of helping governments improve their own national security (including health security) is much lower than that of potential U.S. intervention if those governments fail, and the assistance is more effective.[3]

The Paucity of U.S. Military Health Missions Intended to Build and Sustain Partner Capacity

Despite the importance of health security in countering terrorist and insurgent groups, few military medical operations have been intended to provide it. U.S. military organizations regularly conduct humanitarian missions worldwide, but the vast majority of these missions are dedicated to direct delivery of health care and are often short-lived, one-off projects (particularly outside of Iraq and Afghanistan).[4] In some operations, such as disaster response and joint training exercises, efforts are understandably constrained by budgets, legal authorities, the focus on the immediate needs of the population, and the operational requirements of the military mission. These operations often appear, in a sense, to be misinterpreted as successful capacity building.

The use of MEDCAPs during Operation Iraqi Freedom is a prime example of how health support can be mischaracterized as a success, while in fact it may be an obstacle to capacity building. After the fall of Baghdad in 2003, U.S. Central Command (USCENTCOM) forces routinely conducted MEDCAPs throughout Iraq to assist in stability and reconstruction efforts and as a tool to support local and regional tribal leaders. However, at the height of the counterinsurgency campaign in 2007, operational commanders and some medical personnel reassessed MEDCAPs as being "strategically" ineffective.[5] MEDCAPs were undermining the Iraqi Ministry of Health's institutional responsibilities and crowding out the health services available from local Iraqi caregivers; moreover, they were raising the expectations of the population that the medical care they provided would be available in the future. While the use of MEDCAPs was curtailed and the term fell out of favor in Iraq, the practice continued even as the drawdown of forces began in 2010 (Baker, 2007, p. 70; Cahill, 2009).

Although the efficacy of MEDCAPs in Iraq remains debatable, such operations have been well established in other regions, even if their effects are not well known. Joint Task Force (JTF)–Bravo is a longstanding mission in the U.S. Southern Command that has provided medical support in Honduras since 1983. JTF-Bravo units have routinely conducted medi-

---

[3] In an analysis of the costs of various operations, one RAND report found that "the costs of an intervention skyrocket when U.S. operational units become involved." Moreover, given the cost differential between low-level engagement activities (like BPC-H or other train/equip operations) and interventions like those in Iraq and Afghanistan, "low-level preventive counterinsurgency techniques are cost-effective even when it is extremely unlikely that any given activity or intervention will yield a decisive result" (Vick et al., 2006, pp. 91–92). For example, a set of small engagements that cost $10 million would be worthwhile even if there were a 0.1-percent chance of averting a $10-billion armed intervention.

[4] Even direct health-care operations are often conducted in cooperation and coordination with partner-nation health providers.

[5] See, for example, Baker, 2007, p. 67.

cal operations involving MEDCAPs and medical readiness training exercises (MEDRETEs).[6] These activities have provided medical care to more than 275,000 citizens during 20 years of successful operations. While this strategy has been successful in training U.S. personnel and has provided rudimentary care to Honduran citizens, a comparable level of effort focused on building Honduran health institutions and networks would likely result in a far more enduring capacity—one that eventually would improve governance by Honduran authorities and reduce the need for U.S. personnel.[7]

Finally, in some regions, MEDCAPs and similar operations that have been used are now recognized as insufficient for building partner capacity. Operation Enduring Freedom–Philippines (OEF-P) is often cited as a model for the success of civil-military operations in countering terrorist groups in undergoverned areas. JTF-510, a force led by then–Brig Gen Donald Wurster (USAF), was sent to Basilan Island in February 2002 to separate the Abu Sayyaf group from the population and help the Armed Forces of the Philippines destroy the group. JTF-510 was highly effective in shifting the attitudes and loyalty of local Muslim communities from Abu Sayyaf to the Philippine government and military. Through JTF-510's efforts to facilitate provision of basic health and nutritional needs and pursue high-impact infrastructure projects, the Armed Forces of the Philippines were "able to cultivate closer relations with the people in insurgent-influenced areas" (Wilson, 2006, pp. 7–8).

However, this success was not, until recently, buttressed by simultaneous efforts to build self-sufficient Philippine military and public health capabilities. According to one military observer of U.S. medical operations in the Philippines, MEDCAPs there "are a waste of resources" that could be better utilized to focus on "train[ing] indigenous persons to increase medical capacity, buy them better equipment and let them take care of their own."[8] In 2009, OEF-P leaders and health providers began to develop and conduct medical seminars that sought to overcome some of the shortcomings associated with MEDCAPS (Petit, 2010). By focusing on training, educating, and partnering with the Philippine military and local public health providers before conducting patient care, U.S. forces have taken a supporting role focused on building local capacity and reaching a wider population (Alderman, 2010).

Important USAF and AFSOC Roles in Building Partner Health Capacity

USAF in general and AFSOC in particular can help bridge the gap between guidance for building partners' capacity to provide health security and systematic and sustainable execution. USAF considers building partnerships and partner capacity one of its core functions. The USAF Global Partnership Strategy identifies global partnerships as a strategic end-state for the USAF as follows:

---

[6] MEDRETEs are "U. S. Southern Command–sponsored readiness training exercises designed to provide humanitarian assistance and free medical care to the people of the host nation, while helping improve the skills of U.S. military medical forces and those of military medical professionals of the host nation" (12th Air Force, current as of 2008).

[7] Based on multiple author discussions during 2010–2011 with military and civilian medical experts from Air Force Major Commands (MAJCOMs), other Service component staffs, and NGOs. U.S. medical personnel often value MEDCAPs and other direct-delivery events because they provide experience with ailments and diseases that are not normally encountered in the United States.

[8] Author correspondence with a senior U.S. military officer in the Philippines, November 2009.

Establish, sustain, and expand Global Partnerships that are mutually beneficial. Promoting appropriate civil-military relationships with partner nations is a key element in U.S. Partnerships. Ensuring U.S. partners expand their legitimacy among the populace enhances the mutually beneficial relationship. (U.S. Air Force, 2008, pp. 3–4)

The strategy goes on to emphasize that "increasing the partner capability and capacity allows them to defend their territory, expand the rule of law and governance, and provide support in coalition operations, when appropriate" (U.S. Air Force, 2008, p. 5). It further identifies medical teams as a means USAF offers to building partnerships. These teams "gain access to nations and locations where armed forces would normally be excluded" (U.S. Air Force, 2008, pp. 14–15).

USAF medical personnel are tasked to support GCC theater-engagement strategies around the world. One vehicle for providing this support is the Defense Institute for Medical Operations (DIMO), a joint agency that focuses on disaster preparedness and has provided medical training teams to dozens of countries since its inception in 2002.[9] DIMO's goal is "to become the DoD's focal point for exportable healthcare training" (DIMO, undated, p. 6). It provides teams for site assessments and both resident and nonresident training in disaster planning/consequence management, patient transport/evacuation, disease prevention and management, and health-care policy. The Defense Security Cooperation Agency sponsors courses through the International Military Education and Training and Humanitarian Assistance programs (DIMO, undated, p. 5).

In addition, the International Health Specialist (IHS) program provides 65 active-duty medical professionals to Numbered Air Forces and GCC staffs to serve "as medical consultants and subject matter experts in civil-military medicine, [mission and exercise planners], and . . . medical augmentees when necessary."[10] Aside from their medical skills, IHS professionals provide competency in language and culture, knowledge of regional medical threats and systems, understanding of joint and interagency coordination processes, and the ability to bridge U.S. and coalition medical capabilities. IHS professionals have conducted or participated in numerous subject-matter-expert exchanges, exercises, assessments, and humanitarian assistance/disaster relief (HA/DR) operations. They conduct training in partner nations, focused primarily on disaster response rather than development and governance. IHS provides a small but critical capacity for engaging partners. USAF is the only Service with this kind of established, formal medical program (Huynh, 2010, p. 4).

More generally, MAJCOMs are medical force providers to the GCCs. These medical forces primarily serve in health protection of U.S. forces. Performing this mission successfully requires knowledge of health issues in areas of potential U.S. operation through medical intelligence and health surveillance, knowledge that BPC-H activities can help provide. MAJCOM medical and dental personnel participate in HA/DR operations, MEDCAPs/DENTCAPs and MEDRETEs, exchanges, and other activities where opportunities to build health capacity and relationships in support of DoD and USAF guidance arise. As discussed later, AFSOC

---

[9] DIMO was established in October 2002 when the U.S. Air Force's Institute for Global Health merged with the U.S. Navy's Defense Healthcare Management Institute and then associated in 2003 with the U.S. Air Force School of Aerospace Medicine (DIMO, undated).

[10] Six IHS professionals are available for missions with AFSOC's 6th SOS, which conducts aviation train-advise-assist missions with partners (Huynh, 2010).

has begun developing a systematic approach to building health capacity with foreign partners. Other MAJCOMs could follow suit, particularly in building the capacity of foreign general-purpose forces and, potentially, foreign civil-military endeavors, and they could offer this capability to the GCCs.

In addition to being a USAF MAJCOM, AFSOC is a component command of USSOCOM. Since one of USSOCOM's priorities is to "deter, disrupt, and defeat terrorist threats" (U.S. Special Operations Command, 2010), AFSOC units are organized, equipped, and trained to operate in austere and, at times, "semipermissive" environments like those found in many developing nations. Furthermore, AFSOC advisors are trained to work with disparate, politically sensitive foreign actors, particularly foreign Special Operations Forces (SOFs), many of which are themselves the first elements to venture into their undergoverned regions. AFSOC medical personnel are therefore uniquely suited to conducting BPC-H missions in less-developed nations. Finally, AFSOC is highly capable of marrying partner medical skills and capacity with aviation, which can provide local providers access to remote regions and offers air evacuation capabilities.

Thus, USAF in general and AFSOC in particular are well positioned to emphasize BPC-H in their planning and operations. In some cases, increasing the priority of BPC-H missions (for example, over efforts to build partner capacity for disaster management) in USAF medical training and education could help make additional USAF resources available if and when tasked by combatant commands.

The Potential Need to Define AFSOC's BPC-H Niche

At the time of this study, AFSOC appeared to be one of the few military organizations actively pursuing systematic, sustained BPC-H. As long as its health advisors serve as the "go-to" professionals for this mission, AFSOC's niche is the mission itself. However, as the broader Air Force and the other Services organize, equip, and train U.S. medical, dental, and veterinary assets to conduct BPC-H activities systematically in line with DoDI 6000.16, AFSOC health advisors will need to define a more specific niche for their capabilities within the mission. A number of attributes and capabilities contribute to a future AFSOC niche in health engagement:

- independent operations in austere, semipermissive environments
- small footprint in the partner nation
- expertise working with partner SOFs
- advanced language and transcultural skills
- inculcation of a "BPC mindset" in the medical training pipeline
- broad medical, dental, and veterinary expertise
- dedication to assessment, planning, coordination, and training, with a long-term view of partner capacity
- ability to work with less-developed partner military and civilian establishments, using existing health-care infrastructure
- potential focus on sectors in which other agencies and NGOs are not strong, especially in Africa (e.g., trauma care)[11]

---

[11] Author discussions with international-development experts focused on Africa, April 2010.

- close coordination with AFSOC's 6th SOS to help bring partner aviation to bear in delivery of health services where needed.[12]

AFSOC may seek in the near term to establish BPC-H competencies that complement those brought to bear by other U.S. Special Operations elements, such as the Civil Affairs Brigade in Army Special Forces.

As AFSOC establishes its capability to build partner health capacity for the long term, it may be able to apply useful practices and lessons from other organizations that pursue health and capacity-building efforts in foreign nations. Chapter Three reviews the experiences of several such organizations.

---

[12] Based on multiple author discussions with AFSOC personnel, 2009–2010.

Insights from Other Organizations on Building Partner Capacity

Introduction

This chapter provides observations and insights based on the experiences of other organizations and determines standards of good practice that are applicable to AFSOC's concept for BPC-H missions. Such standards can help AFSOC and the GCCs and TSOCs fashion their own BPC-H models for effective organization, planning, and operations.

Selection of Other Organizations

As noted earlier, AFSOC/SG and RAND selected three organizations from which to gain insights relevant to BPC-H activities: the 95th CA BDE, AFSOC's 6th SOS, and Project HOPE. AFSOC asked RAND to analyze the 95th CA BDE and Project HOPE, and the RAND team suggested the addition of the 6th SOS. Both AFSOC and RAND viewed these organizations as most relevant, given the scope of the project and the experience in which AFSOC was most interested. These organizations had conducted missions that relate to the DoD vision for building partner capacity—a foundation of AFSOC's concept—and they had experience that was valuable to AFSOC. While these organizations were selected for the primary research effort, the RAND team also pursued other experts to provide as broad a review as possible. These experts included current and former military health service professionals with long experience in military medical activities in developing countries and practitioners of development efforts with NGOs. Lessons from these experts are presented later in this chapter, following the discussion of the three selected organizations.

The 95th CA BDE, assigned to the U.S. Army Special Operations Command (USASOC), identifies, plans, and conducts operations that address critical vulnerabilities in designated foreign nations and populations. Though a relatively new organization, the 95th CA BDE was selected because it is a Special Operations unit that conducts health activities in austere environments and contributes to DoD's partnership-building efforts through civil-military engagement (CME) missions.

The 6th SOS was established as an advisory unit in AFSOC in 1994 to train and advise foreign air forces in the employment of airpower for foreign internal defense. For the past 18 years, the 6th SOS has been working to build partner capacity by assessing, training, advising, assisting, and integrating air forces of partner nations, particularly those with less-capable air arms. Though not a unit dedicated to health engagement, the 6th SOS was selected because of its relatively long history of building partner capacity in less-developed nations. Its missions at times have included a health-related element, but this has not been its primary mission focus.

Project HOPE is an NGO founded in 1958 by a former Navy doctor. The Navy donated a ship to Project HOPE that became the first peacetime hospital ship. Since then, Project HOPE has operated in more than 100 countries to strengthen health-care infrastructure, train medical professionals, and provide humanitarian assistance, all key components related to partnership building. Project HOPE was selected because it works with DoD on health-engagement missions and takes a long-term view of capacity building.

Approach to Examining the Three Organizations

Our examination of other organizations included reviewing publicly available information, as well as discussions with organization representatives. The RAND team defined a set of common criteria and related variables, shown in Table 3.1, that would shed light on important practices that AFSOC could apply to its BPC-H planning and execution processes and that would provide bases for comparison among organizations. Several of the criteria (those related to organizational structure and approach) were used for comparing organizations, while others were deemed useful for providing insights into operational effectiveness and lessons learned. Information about each variable was not available for every organization the team examined. Still, the variables allowed for a reasonably systematic review. As AFSOC's BPC-H concept develops, the selected organizations may serve as continuing sources of information about best practices.

95th Civil Affairs Brigade

The 95th CA BDE plays an integral role in both the U.S. Army and DoD as a unit focused on the civil component of military operations. As of July 2010, it was the only active Army brigade conducting CME. Located at Fort Bragg, North Carolina, the 95th CA BDE primarily conducts CME through TSOCs within each of the GCCs. CME is an integrated process in which teams from the 95th CA BDE work with foreign leaders and institutions, as well as selected interagency and intergovernmental partners, to address specified civil issues and needs in designated countries (U.S. Army, 2011). CME missions meet a number of the qualifications for building partner capacity and BPC-H examined in this report.

95th CA BDE Mission and Organization

The 95th CA BDE mission is to "support military commanders by working with civil authorities and civilian populations during peace, contingency operations and war" ("95th CA BDE," 2010). Within this broad mission, Civil Affairs personnel conduct CME to help build partner capacity, gather information, and gain access for other U.S. military forces.

The Army established the 95th CA BDE as the first active-duty Civil Affairs brigade in 2007. This marked a significant change in organizational structure for Civil Affairs, since for the previous 30 years, approximately 95 percent of its units and personnel had been in the Army reserve. However, with continuing mobilizations of reserve Civil Affairs units for deployment to Iraq and Afghanistan, as well as growing demands for support in other contingency operations in such regions as the Horn of Africa and Southeast Asia, a unique, special-

Table 3.1
Criteria and Variables Used to Guide Organization Review

Criterion	Variables Explored
Motivation/mission	Security partnership Economic partnership/investment International disease control Information collection Political Ideological Benevolence/charity
Sponsorship	Military Government, nonmilitary Multiple countries, including host nation Nongovernmental For-profit, nonprofit Command and control relationships
Funding	U.S. Congressional Agency budget (DoD, Department of State, etc.) Multiple countries Foundation or charity (donor funded)
Personnel	Military Nonmilitary Specialties, e.g., medical, dental, veterinary, sanitation, engineering
Mission type	Full-service medical/vet/dental Specific service (e.g., vaccination) Auxiliary service (e.g., sanitation, education)
Duration	Short- vs. long-engagement missions Single vs. multiple missions
Focus	General, engagement with multiple countries Regional (e.g., Central Africa) Single country All peoples vs. specific populations (by age, gender, religion, occupation, etc.)
Training requirements	Trains personnel internally Relies on personnel already trained Also trains personnel in host country
Equipment and logistics	Equipment of other missions (DoD) Dedicated equipment Loaned/donated equipment Host-nation equipment Supplies procured locally or transported Self-reliant logistically Commercial logistics Logistics of convenience/volunteers Ultimate disposition of equipment
Communications	With host-nation government With general population Reach-back capability Public affairs
System to capture mission data and lessons learned	Mission reports After-action briefs
Metrics	Cost Health outcomes Other outcomes (political, economic) Throughput (logistics)

purpose force was needed in the active Army.[1] Currently, the 95th CA BDE has more than 600 personnel assigned in either the brigade headquarters or one of the five subordinate battalions, each of which is designated to support a GCC and its respective TSOC. While the majority of the personnel assigned are Civil Affairs officers and noncommissioned officers, medical support and staffing are substantial, as each battalion has 27 medics, a public health doctor, and a veterinarian ("95th CA BDE," undated).

With their unique focus on supporting both general-purpose forces and Special Forces, Civil Affairs personnel may receive funding for deployment from operations and maintenance in the GCCs, as well as security-forces assistance. When deployed, personnel from the 95th CA BDE conduct operations as task-organized teams supporting military commanders throughout the full spectrum of operations. Teams may be large—e.g., a Civil Military Operations Center with 72 personnel may be used to support civil engagement at the combined- or joint-operations command level. Teams may also be tailored for specific situations—e.g., a Humanitarian Assistance Coordination Center used for disaster response efforts. More routinely, four-person multipurpose teams, identified as Civil Affairs Teams, are deployed from the subordinate battalions in the 95th CA BDE to conduct operations supporting their respective GCC and TSOC. The RAND team reviewed a variation of these smaller Army teams, the Civil Military Support Element (CMSE), which can deploy a modified Civil Affairs Team for capacity-building assessments and missions within a specific country.[2]

In the current operating environment, demand for Civil Affairs support across the GCCs regularly surpasses current capabilities, particularly with the ongoing missions in several countries. Additionally, Civil Affairs units may also be needed for support operations responding to national crises, e.g., Hurricane Katrina in 2005.[3] To meet these demands, the U.S. Army will stand up another battalion, the 85th CA BDE, under USASOC in the next five years.[4]

95th CA BDE Operations and Training

With little more than three years of operational history, the 95th CA BDE has participated in a wide variety of missions, from foreign humanitarian assistance to counterinsurgencies and major combat operations. While many of the missions have involved medical services, including patient treatment, public health assessments, and health logistics, others have focused specifically on BPC in various institutions and communities. This section focuses on CMSE missions that may be characterized as long-term, focused efforts to build partner capacity.

Organizationally, CMSEs employ four or more personnel to work for 30 days to nine months in a partner country. A support team, or "persistent" element, usually composed of two senior Civil Affairs personnel, embeds in the U.S. embassy of the partner country. The operational, or "purposeful," element, comprising four or more Civil Affairs personnel, identifies opportunities for engagement and executes missions.[5] The capabilities of the CMSE operational element may be further enhanced by augmenting team members.

---

[1] For an examination of broader considerations on Army BPC activities, see Marquis et al., 2010, pp. 4–14.

[2] See U.S. Army, 2011.

[3] Civil support operations involve the deployment of Army units, expertise, and capabilities in a domestic environment to support U.S. federal, state, and local authorities.

[4] Provided to RAND by senior Civil Affairs officers from U.S. Army Civil Affairs & Psychological Operations Command on May 15, 2010.

[5] Ibid., p. 8.

While providing medical care for U.S. military personnel remains a first priority for Civil Affairs medics (as it is for AFSOC medics), the medics also routinely provide training for partner-nation military forces, as well as direct care for civilian populations. Medical, dental, environmental, and veterinary services may be provided to achieve a goal (e.g., to protect a population after a flood) or to secure information and access (e.g., to gain access to local leaders and limit the influence of insurgents).

Though CMSEs focus on nontraditional military operations, each mission conducted occurs only after the operational environment has been thoroughly assessed and analyzed using traditional mission-planning tools and techniques. On the basis of standard variables described in both Army and Joint doctrine, such as political, social, and environmental infrastructure, CMSEs acquire thorough background and familiarization on both local and regional communities, their leaders, and their populations' needs. With this preparation and detailed planning, CMSE leaders are able to determine not only how CMSE medical missions will best achieve outcomes in situations with limited time and resources, but also how to link standard reports (e.g., numbers of patients treated during a mission or improved power-generation capacity provided for a local health clinic) to the overall operational plan for engagement within a partner country (U.S. Army, 2008, p. 12).

Medical personnel assigned to the 95th CA BDE are highly trained and equipped for work in austere environments. Each Civil Affairs medic receives eight months of training beyond his or her basic qualifications to develop advanced skills in public health, trauma casualty care, field assessments, and other specialties. During CMSE missions, medics have been key team members for assessing local health facilities and coordinating operations with local health-care providers. Experienced Special Forces officers and noncommissioned officers plan, direct, and coordinate many operations, while licensed doctors, veterinarians, and other providers contribute clinical expertise and evaluation and serve as formal and informal instructors for U.S. and partner forces.[6]

All personnel assigned to the 95th CA BDE receive in-depth cultural familiarization based on their assigned battalions and the associated GCC to which they will deploy and conduct operations. They also receive several months of linguistic training prior to deploying for most missions. This has been a requirement for CMSEs, as the teams remain in a partner country for several months. Additionally, senior Civil Affairs officers and noncommissioned officers are usually selected to lead and staff CMSEs, since their operational experience and maturity are critical for the interaction that is often necessary for successful cross-cultural engagements (Lightsey, 2010, pp. 15–21).

Assessment of 95th CA BDE Activities

Relevant articles, reports, and consultations with CMSE personnel assigned to USCENTCOM, USAFRICOM, and the U.S. Southern Command over the past two years suggest that CMSEs have sought to engage local partners for immediate impact, including identifying and improving the capacity of local authorities to meet the needs of citizens. Feedback from TSOC commanders and local leaders, along with improved public perception of supported partners, has indicated that CMSEs can be successful in gaining access, as well as improving capacity within

---

[6] Fully qualified Civil Affairs medics complete both the Civil Affairs Medical Sergeant Course (6 weeks) and the Special Operations Combat Medic Course (26 weeks) at the John F. Kennedy Special Warfare School and Center (Army Training Requirements and Resources System, 2010).

identified communities. Recent highlights include hospital assessments and population surveys conducted with local leaders after the earthquake in Haiti during Operation Unified Response in 2010 ("Joint Task Force-Haiti Mission Update Brief," 2010); partnering with tribal leaders to improve World Food Program food delivery networks and medical services in the Federally Administered Tribal Areas of western Pakistan under Operation Enduring Freedom in 2009– 2010 (Lightsey, 2010, pp. 21–23); and conducting dozens of missions to train and equip local medical clinics and citizens in Mauritania and Niger under OEF-TS in 2009–2010 (Ward, 2010, p. 26).

Key enablers for CMSEs have been the integrated planning conducted through the TSOC and GCC staffs and the embedded teams linked directly to the U.S. embassy in a partner country. This embedded planning staff allows CMSEs to have greater awareness of other U.S. government efforts in the country and an increased ability to identify opportunities for quick-turn efforts with local authorities and interagency partners, such as expanding the delivery network of the World Food Program. Additionally, CMSEs rely on the doctrinal Civil Information Management process to capture the effects and impact of military support in the civil environment. Constraints on CMSEs include finding suitable partners to accomplish tasks. From recognizing cultural expectations of contracted workers to mitigating excessive demands from local leaders, CMSEs have needed to maintain vigilance and rely on both formal and informal networks to keep communication channels open.

While CMSEs have proved versatile and capable for short-duration capacity-building missions in austere areas, the lasting impact of their efforts is more difficult to assess. When U.S. forces left Haiti after Operation Unified Response relief efforts were complete, wide-scale capacity-building and infrastructure-repair efforts were still under way but had fallen back under the United Nation's Stabilization Mission, and several other U.S. government agencies and NGOs were still supporting the people (U.S. Agency for International Development, 2010a). Haitian government leaders and local officials had never attained the ability to manage or direct these projects independently and were still reliant on foreign support and resources. In western Pakistan, remote tribal communities in the Federally Administered Tribal Areas have routinely suffered from floods, famines, and earthquakes in the past few years, when the population's needs have rapidly overwhelmed even the most well-equipped facilities and hospitals (U.S. Agency for International Development, 2010b). In such communities, with their insufficient infrastructure and weak local governance, one generator for a new community medical clinic or a new schoolhouse will likely have little strategic value in long campaigns to reverse the impact of multiyear disasters and may only temporarily halt the influence of insurgents. Moreover, providing a generator does little to build local capacity in a sustained manner.

Observations on the 95th CA BDE Applicable to AFSOC Health Engagement
In evaluating CMSE efforts to build partner health capacity, there remains the question of whether the CMSEs are engaging in an enduring process. CMSE efforts are only as enduring as military commanders direct them to be. Improving local capabilities requires concerted effort by commanders to maintain momentum and the commitment of time and personnel. Another strategic lesson for AFSOC may be the need to recognize that numerous BPC-H efforts are already ongoing in many partner countries in the health field. Leaders and planners in the 95th CA BDE cited numerous ongoing and past efforts that could be supported in part through CMSEs, including World Health Organization anti-malaria campaigns and national

maternal health requirements for the Millennium Challenge Goals. The challenge may be, as it was for CMSEs, to identify "best-fit" opportunities, given finite resources and time, before committing to a strategy for building capacity.

CMSE experiences provide additional operational lessons applicable to AFSOC's BPC-H concept. First, relationships built between U.S. personnel and partner nations may be more important in the long term than the reported outcomes of any recent mission. CMSE leaders often refer to the trust, confidence, and cooperation that can be built only through multiple engagements that involve positive, transparent communication between U.S. and partner-nation professionals.[7] Many partners reportedly expect this trust and cooperation. Furthermore, understanding U.S. legal and policy constraints may be as important to mission success as learning what partners need and what they can independently manage. This may be simple (e.g., no nine-volt batteries are sold in Pakistan) or complex (e.g., U.S. rules and authorities are not understood by or relevant to tribal leaders or businesses in remote communities), but learning how to bridge institutional gaps within highly synchronized and programmed U.S. military operations can be the most difficult obstacle to providing effective capacity building in a partner country.[8]

U.S. Air Force 6th Special Operations Squadron

The 6th SOS was established as an advisory unit in AFSOC in 1994 to train and advise foreign air forces in the employment of airpower for internal defense. The squadron conducted engagements with partner aviation units, particularly in regions where improvements in capability could support efforts to counter narcotics, as well as terrorist and insurgent groups.[9] Based at Hurlburt Field in Florida, combat aviation advisors (CAAs) of the 6th SOS conduct missions to bring foreign airpower into play in coalition operations. Many of the partner nations with which 6th SOS advisors work field air arms that are significantly smaller and less capable than USAF or the air forces of other developed nations. Moreover, many of the rotary- and fixed-wing aviation platforms and infrastructure CAAs encounter are dissimilar to systems that the United States commonly operates. Initially, 6th SOS advisors concentrated on South American and Middle Eastern countries, but since 2001, their operations have expanded to nearly every region of the world (Moroney et al., 2009, pp. 73–75).

6th SOS Mission and Organization
The mission of the 6th SOS is to "assess, train, advise, and assist foreign aviation forces in airpower employment, sustainment and force integration" (U.S. Air Force, 2010). Its goals are to "bring foreign airpower into play; facilitate host nation aviation availability, reliability, safety, and interoperability; create [a] joint and combined battlefield; [and] support [the] joint force commander" (Air Force Special Operations Command, 2006, pp. 3–4). Advisors conduct tactical training (as opposed to basic flying training) of foreign airmen in a partner nation, using that nation's equipment. The goal is to advance the tactical skills of foreign airmen to enable

---

[7] Author interviews with 95th CA BDE personnel and former CMSE team members at Fort Bragg, N.C., on May 18, 2010.

[8] Ibid.

[9] For an early history of the unit, see Vick et al., 2006, pp. 115–117.

them to operate aviation effectively, conduct joint operations with their nations' ground forces, and ultimately participate in coalition operations with other nations. CAAs seek to use tactical engagements to bring about strategic effects in support of U.S. interests.

Until recently, the squadron comprised only about 100 advisors. Rising demand for their skills, particularly since 2001, led to an increase in their numbers to 207 as of 2010, with further increases planned. Only 145 advisors are assigned, however, and more than half of them were deployed to seven countries at the end of April 2010 (Grub, 2010, p. 4). The 6th SOS is organized into regionally focused flights and operational aviation detachments (OADs), which function as tactical advisory teams attached to the flights. The squadron operates a small number of aircraft at Hurlburt to enable advisors to maintain currency in the platforms (U.S. Air Force, 2010).

The 6th SOS may be tasked to undertake engagements from a number of sources, but the most common sources are the GCCs and TSOCs (through USSOCOM). Often, staff from these commands will contact the 6th SOS directly to inquire about availability of CAAs and will then pursue requests for forces through channels. Categories of operations include Joint/Combined Exchange Training events (JCETs), Joint Chiefs of Staff exercises, Counter-Narcotics Training, and Mobile Training Teams. JCETs, which involve operations and maintenance funds from the unified commands, make up a sizable majority of 6th SOS engagements.[10] The primary purpose of the JCET is to train U.S. service members in general SOF skills and build their region-specific expertise; the benefit to foreign forces is supposed to be incidental.[11]

6th SOS Operations and Training

The CAAs of the 6th SOS have conducted more than 90 missions in 33 countries since 2001. Engagements range from assessments, subject-matter-expert exchanges, and exercises to in-depth tactical training in combat search and rescue, medical evacuation (MEDEVAC), and air-assault operations. In recent years, 6th SOS operations have shifted toward USCENTCOM and USAFRICOM, and CAAs are conducting intensive, longer-term operations in a small number of countries (Moroney et al., 2009, p. 74). For the most part, however, 6th SOS visits to many countries are sporadic. In fact, CAAs visited most of the 33 countries only once (these are often called "one-off" visits), with no follow-on missions,[12] primarily because of changing DoD, GCC, and USSOCOM priorities, an issue addressed below.

CAAs pursue the following general employment concept to build partner aviation capacity:

- *Initiate presence.* A relationship with partner-nation personnel and leaders may be initiated by a visit, which helps the partner understand capabilities the 6th SOS can bring to bear.
- *Assess ground truth.* Assessing ground truth is a key part of the advisory concept, as it helps the advisor understand the partner country's objectives and environment, the status of its aviation capabilities, and its most pressing aviation needs.
- *Train to improve partner-nation tactical skills, safety, and interoperability.* CAAs conduct training in-country on partner-nation platforms and other equipment.

---

[10] Based on a RAND review of 90 missions the 6th SOS conducted between 2001 and 2009.

[11] This is outlined in Title X of the U.S. Code, Section 2011, "Special Operations Forces: Training with Foreign Forces." This is not unlike the purpose of the MEDCAP, which is to help train U.S. medical personnel.

[12] Based on a RAND review of 90 missions the 6th SOS conducted between 2001 and 2009.

- *Incorporate partner-nation capabilities into exercises and contingency operations.* CAAs work with U.S. and partner-nation ground forces to enhance air-ground operations, particularly in less-developed nations where ground forces dominate security institutions.
- *Build partner-nation rapport and confidence.* Advisors seek to ensure sustainment of partner skills through maintenance of personal relationships and repetition of skills.
- *Establish a foundation for combined operations.* CAAs promote capabilities in partner nations that enable those nations to attain interoperability with U.S. and other armed forces, and they seek opportunities to incorporate partner-nation aviation into combined exercises.
- *Advise and integrate capabilities in real-world operations and assist in execution.* CAAs may advise partner aviation units during operations and even assist in mission execution. These activities are conducted less frequently than other parts of the employment concept and are restricted by U.S. law (Air Force Special Operations Command, 2006, p. 22).

Advisors usually deploy in OADs, nominally in groups of 13, although the number varies, depending on the type of engagement. OADs generally include multiple skill sets, including mission commander, pilot, maintainer, communications operator, regional area specialist, force protection, and medic/flight doctor.[13] The average mission length is about 30 days, but in some key countries, missions are significantly longer or may even be continuous. Advisors are sensitive to their cultural environment and may or may not wear military uniforms in-country. Moreover, the OADs are self-contained and have small footprints; support from outside sources while in-country is welcome and often provided by the embassy, the partner nation, or other U.S. forces, but it can be minimal if necessary.[14]

6th SOS personnel are selected from instructor-qualified volunteers elsewhere in AFSOC and the Air Force, and they usually sign up for a four-year tour with the squadron. Upon arrival, personnel initially go through a four-phase, six- to eight-month mission-qualification course. The first 45 days consist of courses at the U.S. Air Force Special Operations School, including courses on cross-cultural communication, regional orientation, international terrorism, and methods of instruction. The next phase, also 45 days, provides integrated skills training, focusing on mission planning, field operations (e.g., small-unit tactics and advanced-weapons employment), and advisor techniques and ends with a "Raven Claw" exercise on combat aviation advising and evasion. Language training comprises the third phase of formal training and lasts from two to four months, depending on the language difficulty. Formal training ends with a one-month focus on survival training and specialty development, during which aircrew and maintainers receive foreign-aircraft initial qualification (Air Force Special Operations Command, 2009). Following formal training, advisors participate in supervised downrange deployments in their focus region. In addition, before any engagement, advisors receive "spin-up" training that includes advanced tactical driving and shooting, communications, medical training, and location-related issues and emergency procedures (Air Force Spe-

---

[13] The 6th SOS has access to six IHS personnel (assigned to the 23rd Air Force at Hurlburt Field) to participate in deployed detachments. The medical element would normally be a supporting activity to an OAD's mission and could involve assessing local medical capabilities and facilities or training foreign military personnel on first aid, buddy care, and other battlefield medical skills. On very rare occasions, deployed IHS personnel may take opportunities to provide basic medical care to local citizens. However, these medical activities do not constitute health-care engagement and are not considered a source of lessons for AFSOC BPC-H activities.

[14] Author discussions with 6th SOS personnel, Hurlburt Air Field, June 22–23, 2009.

cial Operations Command, 2006, p. 20). Beyond this training, advisors are required to maintain language proficiency through classes and on-site interactions with partner nations and to ensure currency in flying and maintaining relevant platforms (Vick et al., 2006, pp. 120–121).

Assessment of 6th SOS Activities

The 6th SOS captures its assessments of partners, lessons, and challenges in standardized mission reports drafted by advisors after each partner engagement. These reports describe the objective of the mission or engagement, the units and personnel involved in the activities, capabilities trained during the engagement, and assessments of the status of the partner's equipment and personnel, challenges faced, and mission outcomes. In cases where the 6th SOS had previously conducted engagements, there is an effort to compare partner capabilities during the current mission with those found previously. Most of the metrics used in the mission reports are qualitative. This is often by necessity, because expert judgment is required regarding the skills foreign airmen have absorbed and whether they have sustained those skills over time. Even more importantly, the relationships forged with partner personnel during these missions are immeasurable, yet critical to U.S. interests.[15]

Overall, a number of key challenges were identified through these reports and through RAND analysis of 6th SOS activities. As noted earlier, many countries are visited intermittently and on an *ad hoc* basis, with little or no follow-through, because the squadron does not control its taskings, which are handed down by USSOCOM in coordination with the TSOCs and GCCs. Priorities regarding countries the squadron is to visit and capabilities to be provided may change from year to year, except for key partners. Moreover, no structured strategy or concept for building partner aviation capacity is broadly accepted across DoD (conversely, medical planning concepts are much more entrenched and accepted across the military medical community). This makes it very difficult to conduct multiyear planning to provide specific capabilities to partners over time. Because missions to individual countries are infrequent, they may be inadequate to build and sustain partner aviation capacity.[16]

The preponderance of JCETs also limits the squadron's ability to build new partner capabilities. Given that JCETs are by law primarily for training U.S. forces and only incidentally for training partner forces, missions must be conducted and assessed based on the benefit to U.S. forces and not on the new capabilities provided to partners. In addition, U.S. law forbids U.S. forces conducting JCETs from leaving U.S. equipment behind with partner forces; thus, advisors cannot provide spare parts to fix broken aircraft that could help accomplish the squadron mission, provide on-the-job training for partner mechanics, and improve partner mission-capable rates.[17] JCETs are not a viable means of building partner capacity by themselves; if combined with other kinds of engagements (such as MTTs), however, they can serve to help sustain partner skills over time.[18]

---

[15] Author discussions with 6th SOS personnel during multiple visits to Hurlburt Field in 2009–2010 revealed a number of cases where long-term relationships have been forged with lower-ranking foreign officers who later became pro-U.S. flag officers and with foreign defense officials. In some instances, these relationships have led to critical support for U.S. operations during times of crisis or conflict. Details of these instances are not releasable to the public.

[16] Based on a review of 90 missions the 6th SOS conducted in 2001–2009 and author discussions with 6th SOS personnel and HQ/AFSOC staff during multiple visits to Hurlburt Field in 2009–2010.

[17] U.S. Code, Title X, Sec. 2011.

[18] Author discussions with 6th SOS personnel and HQ/AFSOC staff during multiple visits to Hurlburt Field in 2009–2010.

Despite these challenges, 6th SOS activities have demonstrated the value of well-trained, experienced advisors who can take advantage of opportunities in uncertain environments characteristic of less-developed regions. Their flexibility and penchant for applying local equipment, skills, and concepts to improve the overall capacity of a partner is unparalleled, especially in countries that offer opportunities for multiple visits. In addition, 6th SOS advisors provide access to and influence with partner-nation decisionmakers (U.S. Air Force, 2009).

Observations on the 6th SOS Applicable to AFSOC Health Engagement

The experiences of 6th SOS combat-aviation advisors provide a number of lessons applicable to AFSOC's BPC-H concept. First, in order to build partner capacity, it is critical to develop and execute multiyear plans for enhancement of specific capabilities in particular countries. In some countries, 6th SOS missions have been hampered by a lack of broadly vetted strategic planning for building aviation capacity at the country and theater levels. However, combat aviation advisors have been extremely successful at executing missions in partner nations, including Colombia, that have benefited from such planning.[19]

Second, multiyear plans should be based on careful assessments of local needs, existing capacity and infrastructure, and other elements of the local environment. They require buy-in from the appropriate theater commands, local partners, other U.S. agencies (especially the country team), and other stakeholders. Such plans also need to take into account other ongoing activities, including civilian efforts (e.g., in the case of building aviation capacity, those taking place under the auspices of the Federal Aviation Administration).

Third, building partner capacity, especially in less-developed nations, requires multiple engagements over a sustained period of time. Countries that have been visited once or twice over the past decade, especially those with marginal existing aviation capability, are not likely to gain BPC benefits.[20] Multiple engagements help build *and sustain* skills and confidence and nurture relationships.

Fourth, AFSOC should work with the tasking GCCs/TSOCs to find a mix of funding sources and tools for its health engagements that facilitate building and sustaining skills over time. Relying solely on JCETs, for example, may not provide the support needed to impart new skills and provide equipment.

Finally, highly trained, experienced, adaptive, and culturally astute professionals enable efforts at the tactical level to be translated into operational and strategic effects. Close working relationships forged by combat-aviation advisors with partner-nation officials have not only enabled improvements in partner aviation capacity but have also provided the United States with access and support in times of crisis and conflict.[21] AFSOC health advisors could likewise enable the United States to benefit in similar ways by applying their training and experience to build effective and sustainable health capacity in less-developed partner nations.

---

[19] See, for example, U.S. Air Force, 2009, p. 6.

[20] There are other tactical reasons for visiting countries only sporadically, including initiating contact with partner militaries and assessing capabilities on the ground.

[21] Author discussions with 6th SOS personnel and AFSOC headquarters staff during multiple visits to Hurlburt Field in 2009–2010; see also U.S. Air Force, 2009.

Project HOPE

Project HOPE was founded in 1958 and has since operated in numerous countries to strengthen health-care infrastructure, train medical professionals, and provide humanitarian assistance. It is a nonprofit organization with a medical doctor as chief executive officer. With few exceptions, members of the board of directors are from private companies, and much of Project HOPE's funding is provided by foundations and companies, through financial contributions or the donation of supplies and equipment. As a nonprofit organization, Project HOPE has a reputation for fiscal responsibility—fundraising and administration account for less than 10 percent of its expenses (based on revenue of approximately $146 million in 2009) (Project HOPE, 2009).

AFSOC's interest in Project HOPE was based on the organization's history of working with the military and conducting long-term health capacity building in the developing world. The RAND team also consulted with other NGOs (discussed in the next section) to ensure that coverage of nonmilitary organizations would be as broad as possible within the scope of the study.

Project HOPE Mission and Approach

The mission of Project Hope is "to achieve sustainable advances in health care around the world by implementing health education programs and providing humanitarian assistance in areas of need." The organization seeks to "provide lasting solutions to health problems with the mission of helping people to help themselves" (Project HOPE, "About Us," undated). It has established working relationships with more than 100 public- and private-sector entities, including the U.S. military; it has worked with the U.S. Navy in 18 humanitarian-assistance missions (including Indian Ocean tsunami relief and Haiti earthquake response) since 2005. It performed a humanitarian mission with the U.S. Air Force in Vietnam in 2009 and helped build a hospital in Basra, Iraq, with the U.S. Army Corps of Engineers, after which it supported hospital operations (HOPE, "Where We Work," undated). It has worked in approximately 100 countries and on every continent since its inception and in 35 countries, including a number of African countries, within the past decade. Project HOPE also publishes the peer-reviewed journal *Health Affairs*.[22]

Project HOPE's efforts generally fall into three categories: medical training and health education, building medical infrastructure, and humanitarian assistance. Much of the humanitarian assistance involves the distribution of donated medical supplies such as pharmaceuticals and vaccines, often in association with companies that not only donate the materials but also provide logistical support—for example, FedEx transported materials for relief in Haiti in support of Project HOPE. Humanitarian-assistance missions are often of relatively short duration, but Project HOPE's long-term focus is on training local health providers, as it has done in programs focused on diabetes education in India, neonatal intensive care in China, and HIV and tuberculosis in Africa (Project HOPE, 2009).

Having a relatively small core staff, Project HOPE relies on volunteers to conduct its work in partner nations. In 2009, 100 Project HOPE volunteers provided health services to more than 100,000 patients and provided training to 40,000 local health-care workers worldwide;

---

[22] See *Health Affairs*, "About the Journal," 2010.

more than 400 volunteers responded to the tsunami in Southeast Asia in 2005 (Project HOPE, 2009).

Assessment of Project HOPE Activities and Observations Applicable to AFSOC Health-Care Engagement

RAND's review of Project HOPE focused on publicly available documents and consultations with a senior Project HOPE official. The documents provided a view of the organization's finances, associate relationships, and activities. There was no indication that Project HOPE conducts detailed assessments of its missions beyond tracking input measures such as the amount of medicine distributed, donations received, and number of health-care workers trained (Project HOPE, "Financial Information," undated). Such measures can be used for advocacy but may provide only part of what is needed to evaluate existing processes or improve mission execution.

The document review and discussions provided some observations worth further consideration. Unlike most military health operations, Project HOPE takes a long-term view of engagement, providing immediate humanitarian assistance in some cases but also conducting much lengthier campaigns—on the order of years—to improve health care in partner countries through education and infrastructure improvements. By contrast, most military health missions are of short duration. This can lead to confusion or frustration in the host country, as short engagements may raise expectations of future assistance that is not offered. When DoD is not able to provide a sustained presence or make multiple visits to a particular country, an associate organization might provide such a presence between military BPC-H missions.

Associations between organizations conducting BPC-H—for example between DoD (or AFSOC) and NGOs—might enable longer-term strategic planning. Longer planning horizons, perhaps five years, could provide mutual benefit to DoD and its associates. Some NGOs rely primarily on volunteers to conduct missions, some of whom might be willing to staff military BPC-H missions. A longer planning horizon would permit the military to count on such staff augmentation and provide the time for its associate NGO to arrange for it. Similarly, an associate organization, given sufficient planning notice, might better arrange for the donation of supplies and equipment from other organizations in support of military BPC-H. Memorandums of understanding might codify such relationships and reduce uncertainty for both military planners and their nonmilitary counterparts.

Observations on Other Organizations

In addition to reviewing the 95th CA BDE, the 6th SOS, and Project HOPE, RAND held discussions with other governmental organizations and NGOs that provided useful insights about BPC-H and other forms of partner engagement. The RAND team used the criteria and variables listed in Table 3.1 to guide discussions with experts in military health and international development to broaden the sources of insight from which AFSOC health advisors might benefit. Interlocutors included officials engaged in health policymaking and planning in the Office of the Secretary of Defense, theater commands (in particular, USEUCOM, USAFRICOM, and SOCAFRICA), other USAF health-related organizations (including IHS and DIMO), and the U.S. Army; and officials from the World Bank and the Academy for Educational Development. Insights from these discussions are relevant to AFSOC for at least two reasons: (1) other DoD organizations are considering some version of health engagement, and AFSOC will likely be working with many of them to build partner health capacity; and (2) the NGO experts have extensive experience in less-developed countries.

This section summarizes the insights of officials at these other organizations and provides relevant citations to the development literature. The following seven observations are particularly applicable to AFSOC efforts to build partner health capacity.

First, *it is important to understand the political, economic, cultural, social, and historical context of a host country.* This involves identifying the major players in and champions of the engagement mission, including senior government officials, bureaucrats, local leaders, and the local medical community. The goal is to gain insight into their main needs, interests, and expectations and why they may support or oppose the enterprise.

Second, *it is equally important to involve the U.S. ambassador, other U.S. officials (e.g., the USAID country chief), and foreign organizations that may also be engaged in the country, such as NGOs.* Effective approaches to such involvement have included "whole-system-in-one-room sessions," where all the stakeholders meet regularly to promote trust in and transparency of the health engagement process. This process may also highlight niche areas, such as veterinary care or treatment of diseases, in which BPC-H could provide value that is not otherwise provided by the local community or other BPC-H organizations.[23]

Third, *successful efforts to build indigenous capacity take into account the available local medical capacity and its potential for augmentation or expansion.*[24] For example, providing equipment that cannot be supported technically or that requires a reliable power supply where none is available can ultimately undermine the best intentions of the donating organization. Similarly, a large or rapid influx of resources into a community that is not equipped to manage them because of a lack of either expertise or supporting infrastructure may result in the waste of those resources or, in some cases, may lead to corruption.[25]

Fourth, *the more BPC-H missions build on or expand local capacity to create immediate benefits for a large number of people, the more likely those missions are to gain local buy-in.* Health-engagement missions that replace local capacity may in fact distance potential local champions of the effort, as happened with the MEDCAPs in Iraq. In some cases, local capabilities may be expanded for immediate and significant benefit. This has been experienced with essential services such as water and electric power, social services, community development, education, and particular medical services that were previously unavailable locally.[26]

Fifth, *it is important to involve local authorities and professionals throughout the entire planning and implementation process.* Not only does such involvement promote local support of the BPC-H mission, it can also help to encourage realistic expectations of the benefit of the mission. As the mission evolves, this involvement can help to adjust expectations when further information is available, such as information about the local absorptive capacity, and it can help to identify opportunities for further—or different—intervention strategies that can become "quick wins" or can provide a significant return on the mission investment. Involvement of local officials should be based on frequent and transparent communication

---

[23] See also Cariappa, Mohanti, and Bonventre, 2008.

[24] See also Parr et al., 2002, pp. 61–84; Rowe et al., 2010; Sun and Marc, 2008.

[25] See also Bhargava, 2006; Rowe et al., 2010, p. 5.

[26] See also Tang et al., 2005; Parr et al., 2002; Rowe et al., 2010, pp. 5–6.

to build trusting relationships between the BPC-H organization, local caregivers, and the local population. Frequent and consistent documentation of mission activities, successes, and obstacles can further promote communication, particularly when the credit for successes can be shared with the host nation.[27]

Sixth, *the most successful BPC-H missions involve sustained interaction with local communities and caregivers in a manner that builds long-term capacity in the local health community.* As one official noted, BPC-H "is a marathon, not a sprint." Anecdotal evidence suggests that some international health efforts have been counterproductive, because they provided short-term medical care to a local population that expected continuing care that was subsequently unavailable. To be successful, BPC-H missions should provide improved care, enhanced infrastructure, trained caregivers, and health education to the population. Whatever the terms of engagement, it is important to articulate a clear exit strategy, explaining when the BPC-H mission will end and what short- and long-term benefits can be expected by the partner nation.[28]

Finally, *it is important to consistently use well-defined metrics and indicators to promote and define long-term success.* Many medical missions employ process or output metrics, such as the number of patients treated or supplies provided. Measurements of improved capacity, while more difficult to quantify, can provide a more accurate picture of success. A strategic approach is most desirable, with a focus on gathering information that will help to sustain long-term support and funding for the mission and attain mission objectives. Such an approach could include process measurements in the near term (number of medical personnel trained), outcome measurements in the mid-term (number of patients treated), and capacity-building measurements in the long term (improvements in health-providers' number and quality, and sustainable infrastructure, for example).[29]

Summary

Reviews of the 95th CA BDE, the 6th SOS, and Project HOPE produced several observations and insights for AFSOC's consideration, and discussions with other organizations complemented or supplemented these observations. First, continuing to improve partner capabilities requires concerted effort over the long term to enhance specific capabilities in particular countries. Most military health missions to date have been of short duration; this can lead to confusion or frustration in the host country by raising expectations of future assistance that is not offered. Second, partnership among all relevant stakeholders conducting BPC-H and involving local caregivers may benefit from longer-term strategic planning by GCCs, NGOs, and partner countries and the application of well-defined metrics. A multiyear planning horizon with multiple engagements and a clearly articulated exit strategy could result in mutual benefit to DoD, its associates, and, ultimately, partner nations. Finally, it is important to recognize that BPC-H efforts are already ongoing in many of the partner countries and to identify "best-fit" opportunities.

---

[27] See also Hartwig, Humphries, and Matebeni, 2008; Hale, 2008, pp. 7–19; Rowe, 2010, pp. 5–6.

[28] See also Tang et al., 2005, pp. 285–295; Rowe et al., 2010, pp. 5–6.

[29] See also Jones et al., 2006; Hartwig, Humphries, and Matebeni, 2008, pp. 251–259.

The next chapter defines a conceptual framework for planning, executing, and assessing BPC-H activities, based on AFSOC's approach and observations of the practices of other organizations.

CHAPTER FOUR

A Framework for Planning and Executing Missions to Build Partner Health Capacity

This chapter presents a conceptual framework and develops generic metrics to support AFSOC health engagement. GCC, TSOC, and AFSOC pursuit of BPC-H occurs within a political and institutional context that is defined by national and theater security cooperation priorities and objectives, and appropriate metrics can help inform internal planning, resourcing, coordination, monitoring, and evaluation. Such metrics can also help communicate progress and achievements to external audiences in DoD, other federal agencies, governmental and nongovernmental entities in partner nations, local communities in partner nations that stand to benefit from BPC-H, and organizations that are active in international health and economic development with whom AFSOC and theater commands might associate.

We begin with a general discussion of metrics and the assessment of effectiveness. Then, a conceptual framework is developed for GCC, TSOC, and AFSOC planning and assessment of BPC-H activities. This framework offers a phased approach to measuring success in conducting BPC-H and suggests examples of metrics that are relevant to potential BPC-H missions.

Metrics and Assessment of Effectiveness

While businesses typically focus on efficiency in assessments, since their bottom line is measured in dollars, effectiveness often is a more important concern for governments when the overarching goal is the delivery of public goods: national security, public safety, justice, health, and social welfare.[1] The following discussion addresses how metrics can be useful for BPC-H assessment.

Measuring Effectiveness and Understanding Its Challenges

Metrics provide important information on how effectively an organization is achieving its objectives as well as how efficient its processes are in supporting those objectives. In business, a basic distinction between efficiency and effectiveness is that the former is typically a measure of time (e.g., the number of minutes it takes to produce a widget from start to finish), while the latter is a measure of quality (e.g., the number of widgets that fail to meet production standards). With the aid of appropriate metrics, their supporting measures (standards as a basis for

---

[1] The push for improved government performance and accountability resulted in the passage of the Government Performance and Accountability Act (GPRA) in 1993. GPRA expands reporting requirements for federal agencies with the use of metrics as a central component. See U.S. Government Accountability Office (undated) for information on implementation of GPRA by various federal agencies.

comparison, such as time, length, temperature, speed), and associated indicators (e.g., using numbers to measure time, sensors to detect motion, chemicals that change color when exposed to heat to monitor change), a business can learn what works and what does not to improve operations, better align resources, motivate personnel, and highlight successes to superiors and other important audiences (Hauser and Katz, 1998; U.S. Government Accountability Office, 2005).

For activities and programs that relate to delivery of public goods, assessing effectiveness can be more challenging because not only are a program's outputs (e.g., number of health workers trained) of interest, the outcomes that align with the objectives of the effort (e.g., improved community access to health services) are as well. A logic chain can help to elucidate relationships between inputs such as money and personnel for activities, outputs (e.g., new health workers), factors that may affect execution of activities, success in producing outputs and their use (e.g., eligible recruits available and license requirements), and, ultimately, the ability to achieve intended outcomes (e.g., improved community health).[2]

Assessment of Effectiveness for Military Health Engagement

Assessing the effectiveness of an activity is ultimately tied to the activity's goals (Kirby, 2005; National Partnership for Reinventing Government, 1999; U.S. Government Accountability Office, 2005). AFSOC's concept for BPC-H is to link its efforts not only to military objectives or end states, but also to those activities that international-development and health experts broadly agree can help produce direct and important benefits to a developing nation's capacity to deliver health services. Such activities include increasing the medical readiness of military forces, as well as improving the health of civilian populations (maternal health services, infectious disease prevention, basic hygiene and sanitation education, etc.).[3]

If increasing the number of trained personnel and the availability of appropriate equipment was the goal of AFSOC's BPC-H concept, then output metrics that measure the number of persons trained to provide health care and to operate associated equipment would be sufficient. However, considering that the goals more broadly are to increase partner-nation capacity to meet public health needs, build a more positive image of the local government and of the United States, strengthen nation-to-nation ties, and generally reduce the vulnerability of local populations to insurgent and terrorist groups, assessing the achievement of objectives will require more than measuring the outputs of BPC-H activities.

Rather, by assessing the *effectiveness* of BPC-H activities, tasking commands should be able to demonstrate how efforts relate to and support broader goals and how the outputs of the activities—i.e., trained personnel and maintained equipment—can help bring about desired outcomes. Consequently, measures that link inputs to outputs and outcomes (means to ends) must take into consideration how BPC-H activities contribute to building partner capacity and

---

[2]   Said another way, "Outputs are the products of program activities, outcomes are the changes resulting from the projects" (Moroney et al., 2010). In DoD parlance, outputs are assessed through measures of performance, while outcomes are assessed through measures of effectiveness. See Haims et al., 2011, p. 10; McCawley, 1997.

[3]   Research calling for attention to BPC in health includes work by Krueger (2008) and Hale (2008). Both highlight the potential benefits of U.S. military efforts to improve health capacity in partner nations, including improving the health of host-nation populations, reducing their sense of disenfranchisement, reducing dependency on foreign agencies, and making extremism less attractive. They also caution that emphasis must be on building capacity of local institutions rather than replacing their health services with direct care by U.S. forces and that it is important to be aware that building capacity is a long-term endeavor.

the attainment of other goals in a complex environment. In other words, metrics are needed that link the U.S. investment to a vision of BPC in the long term and achieving key U.S. objectives in a theater, subregion, or partner nation.[4]   Thus, before metrics are developed, the outcomes and associated inputs and outputs that enable achievement of these objectives must be defined. With this information, GCCs, in concert with USAID and other agencies, can begin planning a BPC-H mission or program and tasking subordinate units to provide the necessary capabilities.

Selecting Assessment Metrics for BPC-H Activities

Once the inputs, outputs, and outcomes are defined, the first step in selecting the right metrics for assessing the mission is determining what AFSOC and the theater elements it supports need to know in order to monitor and implement BPC-H plans in a given partner nation or region. Metrics should be actionable in terms of informing decisions and operations throughout the life cycle of a program, including

- during strategy development and planning to identify and test assumptions and hedge against their failure
- during implementation of an operation or program to track progress and adapt to new conditions
- after completion of the mission or program, to evaluate impact and draw lessons.[5]

Metrics are needed that can help AFSOC and the GCCs/TSOCs it supports to communicate effectively that they are performing their activities relative to the stated goals or desired outcomes. Metrics (as well as qualitative evaluations) should be used to show how military BPC-H activities contribute to improved health and security conditions in high-risk areas, expanded U.S. military ties with indigenous elites, and perhaps enhanced technical and cross-cultural training opportunities for USAF and other military personnel, in addition to demonstrating increased partner-nation capacity in public health (Brown, LaFond, an McIntyre, 2001; National Partnership for Reinventing Government, 1999).

Finally, quality of metrics matters far more than quantity. Keeping the number of metrics to the minimum necessary to measure only the inputs, outputs, and outcomes required to achieve stated objectives helps planners and assessors, avoids clutter, and sharpens focus. Collecting, collating, and maintaining data can incur considerable financial and labor costs (U.S. Government Accountability Office, 2005). Thus, the number of metrics should be kept to the minimum needed to support budget and management decisions; inform superiors and important audiences about progress toward achieving objectives; and motivate partners, associates, and supporters.

With this general discussion of metrics as background, we next define a conceptual framework for planning health-engagement efforts. Metrics for BPC-H activities will then be identified in the context of this framework.

---

[4] Several constructs have been developed to link means to ends. See, for example, Thaler, 1993; Haims et al., 2011.

[5] See Kirby, 2005; U.S. Government Accountability Office, 2005.

Conceptual Framework: A Phased Approach to BPC-H Efforts

This section develops a four-phase conceptual approach to planning for, implementing, and assessing the effectiveness of a health engagement activity. The approach is based on numerous discussions in spring and summer 2010 with civilian and military professionals who have experience in international health work, as well as a review of the literature on international development.[6] Although AFSOC and theater BPC-H activities will generally involve multiyear efforts in specific health sectors within individual partner nations, this approach could also be applied to regional efforts. Input, process, output, and outcome metrics help monitor alignment of implementation with goals and strategy during the four phases of the framework, which are

1. consult, plan, and prepare for start-up
2. launch activities
3. conduct full-scale implementation
4. draw down, transition, and (possibly) withdraw.

This conceptual framework correlates well with AFSOC's concept for health engagement in that it proposes an end-to-end, systematic approach to planning and implementing BPC-H missions to attain desired outcomes.

Figure 4.1 shows the framework in a hypothetical multiyear BPC-H effort in a partner nation. Each phase is defined by the major action(s) that U.S. military health advisors and tasking theater commands, along with associated agencies and organizations, would need to undertake to achieve the goals of the effort. The curves in Figure 4.1 show heuristically the level of involvement in executing a training activity over time for AFSOC (and other tasked military organizations) and tasking theater commands and associates and/or the partner nation. This is one of a number of ways a BPC-H program could be executed over time. In this case, the U.S. military and other agencies (e.g., USAID) are heavily involved in organizing, planning, and implementing the program, in coordination with partner-nation authorities and/or associate organizations (e.g., NGOs). At the beginning, the U.S. commands and agencies provide the bulk of the planning and training capacity. While the partner is fully integrated for planning and coordination, its capacity is not yet developed. As the partner and/or associate increases its contribution to the activity, the U.S. military scales back its own participation.

At some point, U.S. military health advisors hand over leadership and ownership of the activity to the partner and/or associate and greatly reduce U.S. involvement (without necessarily reducing interest in tracking future outcomes). This case is merely illustrative; levels of involvement over time (and thus the shapes of the lines) could be drastically different, depending on the situation. Other examples could depict high levels of partner involvement in training activities from the beginning or varying levels of U.S. and partner involvement over the course of the program.

---

6   See Malsby, 2008; Baker, 2007; Bricknell and Thompson, 2007; Cariappa, Mohanti, and Bonventre, 2008; Wilder, 2009.

Figure 4.1
Framework for a Hypothetical BPC-H Training Program

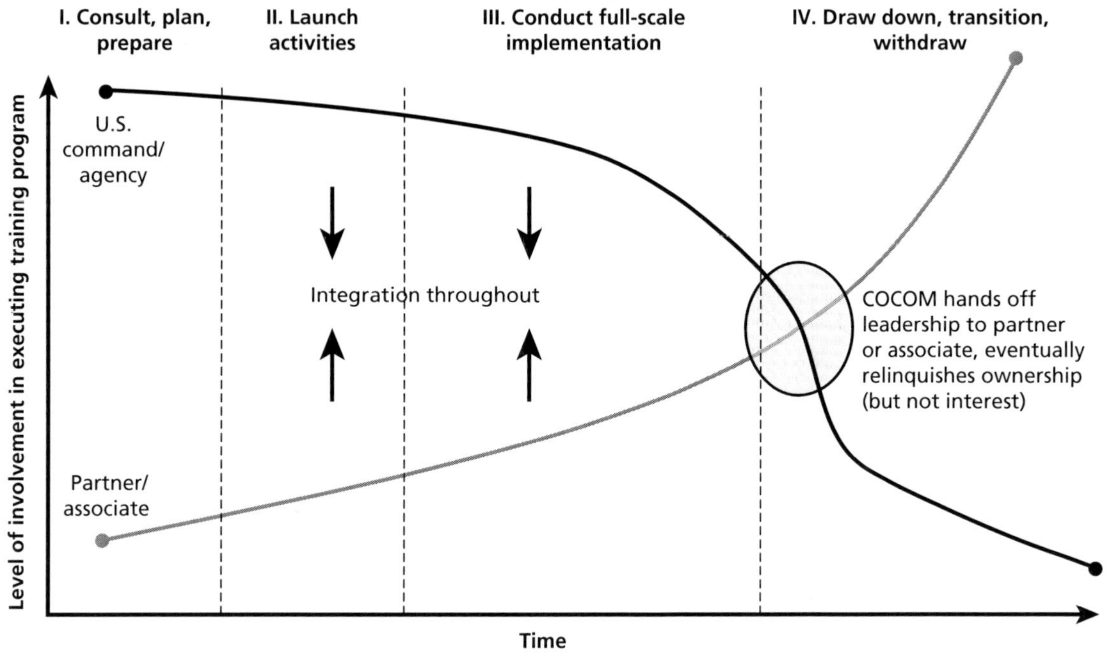

Phase I: Consult, Plan, and Prepare for Start-Up

The central activity in the first phase of the framework is theater command and AFSOC inter-facing with the partner nation, relevant U.S. embassy personnel and other U.S. agencies, and potential associates to assess local health-care needs, understand the local environment, iden-tify appropriate activities, plan, and harness the necessary funds, staff, space, transportation, equipment, and curricula for the BPC-H effort. The health and international-development experts consulted in this study highlighted success in using multiday consultation events that bring together important stakeholders to review plans, approaches, and metrics. Such forums allow airing of various viewpoints, illuminate critical assumptions, highlight important stake-holders that are missing, and facilitate reconciliation of differences. Even absent such events, deliberate and careful consultation with important stakeholders is paramount.

In the example shown in Figure 4.1, AFSOC and other military health advisors are deeply involved at the inception of the BPC-H activity. Metrics at this stage should help planners con-firm the validity of the plan and ensure that the right stakeholders are on board and the right resources are applied.

Phase II: Launch Activities

When the plans, approach, resources, and agreement of important entities are confirmed, the BPC-H activities can be launched, e.g., training the partner-nation military medical corps (and possibly civilian health workers), providing equipment, and/or upgrading health facilities and infrastructure.[7] Health advisors might conduct pilot activities to test the waters, learn, revise plans and processes, and reallocate resources as appropriate to prepare for full-scale implementation. Metrics in this phase would monitor progress and document lessons learned to provide data for analysis to determine whether the BPC-H effort is ready for full-scale implementation.

The first two phases might be completed relatively quickly, e.g., within the first year of a three- to four-year program. Still, it is necessary to invest time and resources in these two phases to create a solid foundation for full-scale implementation and to sustain the effort in the long term.

Phase III: Conduct Full-Scale Implementation

Full-scale implementation gets under way in the third phase. In the case shown in Figure 4.1, the partner or associate assumes a greater role in management and implementation, while the level of U.S. military involvement declines. Metrics would not only monitor progress of activities but would also assess how well the partner or associate is performing in its expanded role. Metrics should also gauge whether the partner has the commitment, the personnel, and the potential to harness sufficient resources to take over the BPC-H effort in the final stage. If the partner fails to perform well in this phase, plans may need to be revised. Also, data collected on partner or associate performance would help the theater commands and AFSOC report progress to important audiences and obtain input on preferred courses of action—for example, on how to alter the program to obtain improved partner performance and/or commitment.

Phase IV: Draw Down, Transition, and Withdraw

In the final phase of the framework, leadership of the BPC-H effort transitions from the U.S. military and other agencies to the partner nation or an associated stakeholder (e.g., an NGO), especially when the program must be sustained until the partner has adequate capacity to assume it. Hand-over could occur early in this phase to allow time for the theater command to confirm that the program can be sustained with minimal or no U.S. military involvement. Without some assurance that the partner can effectively sustain the effort after the departure of U.S. military and civilian health advisors, the BPC-H effort could fail to build sustainable partner health capacity. In alternative cases where an associate or partner performs the bulk of the training activity early in the process, the military handoff may relate to specific elements of a program.

The framework makes a distinction between ownership and leadership, based on their differing roles. Here, ownership primarily involves providing and overseeing resources for a BPC-H activity and having a say in the strategic goals of the effort. Ownership organizations include grant-making foundations and federal grant programs, which provide resources for projects but are not necessarily involved in the daily operation or implementation of activities. Leadership involves running the day-to-day operation, developing a vision and plans to achieve strategic goals and objectives, implementing activities to achieve these goals and objectives, and conducting analysis to report on progress and achievements.[8] An organization with leadership responsibilities may provide funding (its own or from outside sources), or it may be contracted to operate a program and execute its activities.

---

[7]   At the time of this study, AFSOC was focusing its efforts on providing training and equipment, not on upgrading facilities, a task for which other U.S. military organizations might be better suited.

[8]   This is analogous to the roles of the owner of a professional football team (ownership) and the coach (leadership).

A U.S. agency (the U.S. military, USAID, or some other agency) could choose to stay involved as the "owner" after the initial launch and operation of a BPC-H activity. It might provide funding as well as oversight and mission guidance to sustain the BPC-H effort after it is handed over to the partner. A number of the experts consulted in this study pointed out that this would be important if the partner cannot clearly show stable commitment of financial resources to sustain the health-care effort. In addition to possibly wasting the initial U.S. investment in the effort, collapse of the activity could tarnish the image of the United States and its military forces in the eyes of the partner government and the image of the partner government in the eyes of its citizens.

Similarly, to help sustain the BPC-H effort under new leadership, the United States (and possibly even the country team) might consider providing critical expertise or equipment periodically. Such involvement would help ensure that newly trained personnel, enhanced equipment, and facility upgrades could take root to effect improved health outcomes. It would also allow U.S. health advisors to directly observe progress on the ground and maintain relationships with important individuals and organizations in the partner nation.

Developing Metrics in the Context of the Framework

At the time of this study, USAFRICOM and SOCAFRICA were implementing programs to build health capacity in OEF-TS countries and elsewhere in Africa.[9] For this initial foray into BPC-H, U.S. military medical personnel are to conduct periodic two- to five-day courses in a medical skill for military personnel from one or more OEF-TS countries. The goal is to train more local caregivers, which will provide expanded access to skilled health care, particularly in rural communities that are undergoverned and have very limited access to transportation and hospitals.

We have developed generic metrics for each phase of a BPC-H program as portrayed in the conceptual framework to help guide definition of more-specific metrics for use in planning and implementing future programs under consideration in Africa and elsewhere.

In the efforts being pursued by USAFRICOM, SOCAFRICA, and AFSOC, the local military is the partner that will assume long-term leadership of the program when the U.S. military has trained a large enough cadre of trainers to sustain the selected medical skill without AFSOC or other U.S. military involvement. At the same time, local civilian government agencies, especially health and finance ministries, are also seen as potential partners. Their participation in a BPC-H effort would enable long-term sustainment of health capacity by supporting future train-the-trainer activities to encourage adoption of new medical techniques throughout targeted OEF-TS countries, particularly in their undergoverned areas.

Table 4.1 summarizes the generic metrics recommended for each phase of the BPC-H effort. Each metric can be supported by a variety of qualitative and quantitative measures and indicators. The metrics are associated with the goals of the BPC-H effort and are designed to enable the U.S. military to monitor, assess, and report progress, performance, and successes throughout the life cycle of the effort. The particular measures and indicators for each metric may change over time as better ones become available. For example, the level of need for emergency obstetrics (Metric 1) could be measured by data on maternal mortality, with high mor-

---

[9] The type of medical skill upon which local military medics will be trained has not been determined.

Table 4.1
Generic Metrics for the Four Phases of a BPC-H Effort

I. Consult, Plan, Prepare	II. Launch Activities	III. Conduct Full-Scale Implementation	IV. Draw Down, Transition, Withdraw
Metric 1: Level of need for effort	Metric 5: Adequacy of contact points and regular consultations	Metric 9: Effectiveness and efficiency of processes	Metric 12: Readiness for hand-over
Metric 2: Level of broad endorsement from superiors and important audiences	Metric 6: Level of success in recruiting trainees and conducting training	Metric 10: Results of immediate outputs and intermediate outcomes over time	Metric 13: Level of benefit to the partner nation and the United States
Metric 3: Development of hedging options	Metric 7: Level of partner performance	Metric 11: Impact on U.S. military training and access	
Metric 4: Level of resource adequacy to execute effort	Metric 8: Readiness to scale up		

tality rates serving as a strong indicator of need. Another measure—a qualitative one—may be the expressed desire of a local government to receive international assistance to reduce high maternal mortality rates as a way to improve social and economic well-being in rural communities (Metric 2).

Generic Metrics for Medical Training in Phase I

The major activities in Phase I of our example are assessing and understanding the social, economic, and cultural environment in and challenges facing rural trans-Sahel communities and evaluating the ability of local and national authorities to provide health care. These activities would focus on the need for access to particular types of medical care and the skills to be targeted for improvement. The U.S. theater commands, in coordination with U.S. embassies and local governments and militaries, would identify a partner nation in which to develop a program and goals for building capacity in a new medical skill. U.S. military health advisors would help identify stakeholders, particularly NGOs and other organizations with which the advisors and the local government might associate. Local military units that are to receive training from U.S. military health advisors would be identified. Importantly, resources must be secured to implement engagements over time.

Metric 1: Level of need for the BPC-H effort. Having an environment that is receptive to the BPC-H effort is critical to success. It is necessary to assess the political, security, cultural, ethnic, and medical conditions in the areas where new skills might be applied. What is the most important unaddressed health-care issue facing the targeted community? What are the community's cultural and ethnic compositions and how do they translate into the way it interacts with the outside world? To whom do members of the community owe allegiance and why? Who provides local health-care services, if any, and what is their capacity? What NGOs already work in the area, and what are they doing? These questions and many more need to be addressed before any BPC-H activity can be planned.

Once these questions are answered and a critical medical need is identified and targeted, the next step is to develop an appropriate plan. Measures and indicators to evaluate the appropriateness of the plan may include articulation of the strategy, timeline, activities, resource requirements, and partner and associate entities, as well as the critical assumptions of the plan.

Metric 2: Level of broad endorsement from superiors and important audiences. Except for the endorsements from relevant U.S. military and civilian agencies, the most important endorsements for any BPC-H effort are those from the local military and ministry of health (which may have authority over health matters, including approval to use certain medical techniques and drugs). Such endorsements are the measures, and indicators for them may be signed agreements or official memorandums and policy statements, as well as verbal agreements by traditional elders before tribal councils. U.S. health advisors would need to consult directly or through SOCAFRICA, USAFRICOM, and the U.S. embassy with partner government offices responsible for rural development activities, because these offices are important allies in expanding the use of new techniques where they are most needed in the country. Consultation with multilateral development banks and international and local NGOs working on health capacity building in the partner nation is also desirable, if not essential. These organizations, too, can be allies in helping U.S. advisors and local military personnel gain access to important community leaders and institutions (e.g., tribal elders and local administrators) whose support is critical to achieving the goals of the BPC-H effort.

Through these development and health groups, U.S. military advisors and local military medical personnel can learn how best to identify future trainees, recruit them, and insert new techniques into the indigenous health landscape. In sum, conducting deliberate consultation to obtain formal and informal endorsements from important audiences inside the U.S. government and in the partner nation may be especially important for building positive relationships and projecting a positive image of the local government and of U.S. presence.

Along with these formal and informal endorsements, another set of indicators is a checklist of all the important audiences identified, with notations as to who endorsed the BPC-H effort and who objected to it and why. The latter information can be important for alerting U.S. advisors about potential obstacles and seeking ways to respond to them.

Metric 3: Development of hedging options. All plans are developed with assumptions, and assumptions are not foolproof. Thus, it is important to have a Plan B ready in case Plan A (the base plan) fails to win acceptance or fails in practice. Having hedging options for critical assumptions in the base plan will help advisors anticipate and prepare for actions to ensure the BPC-H effort can move forward even if significant changes occur in the environment, e.g., loss of a major associated organization (Dewar et al., 1993). Good plans always allow a level of flexibility to adapt to and succeed in changing conditions.

For example, USAFRICOM may assume that local military personnel would welcome the opportunity to learn a particular medical skill and would be able to conduct train-the-trainer activities. However, the local military personnel may have a high turnover rate, indicating that trained personnel may not stay around long enough to extend new techniques to civilian first responders and caregivers. Also, the theater command must ascertain whether civilian first responders and caregivers are motivated to learn the new techniques even when there is no monetary reward for knowing more and doing more. Finally, caregivers may have had previous experiences in which they did not have a stable supply of drugs or medical supplies for use in new treatment procedures.

These are everyday realities that international-assistance participants must consider in many developing countries, including those in Africa. Working with multilateral development banks and bilateral aid agencies, the GCC/TSOC and the U.S. embassy could attempt to persuade the partner nation's finance ministry to allocate more aid dollars to the health ministry. Multilateral development banks and bilateral aid agencies can also be allies in promoting improved governance among organizations involved in the BPC-H effort. Again, considering that the initial BPC-H effort would be small in a landscape filled with many players, identifying critical assumptions and having hedge options for them would help the theater commands succeed.

Importantly, planners may also need to hedge against changes in U.S. military priorities. Hedging options should account for potential crises in other parts of the world that take BPC-H–tasked health advisors away from these efforts and render them unavailable for periods of time.

For this metric, measures are the critical assumptions, and the indicator is a list of those assumptions, with clear articulation of why they are critical and what could happen to the implementation and success of the BPC-H effort if the assumptions prove faulty. For example, if the assumption that local first responders and caregivers want to learn from local military personnel is incorrect, one option might be to involve local leaders in efforts to understand and address their lack of interest. Another option might be to invite the leaders, first responders, and caregivers to observe the U.S. training of the local military personnel in the new medical techniques and explain what is involved. Still another option might be to have first responders and caregivers who have received the training, as well as the local leaders and beneficiaries of the training (e.g., in the case of emergency obstetrics, new mothers and their spouses), visit other towns or regions to share their positive experiences.

Metric 4: Level of resource adequacy to execute the BPC-H effort. This metric is a simple one. The central issue is whether the funds, manpower, equipment, and other resources needed consistently over time will be secured to fully implement the effort.

Measures may consist of numbers of personnel, amount of funding, and number and type of equipment needed and available. Indicators may include data that show the amount of resources that can be harnessed vis-à-vis what is required in the plan. Data collected should indicate whether the requisite resources have been obtained to move forward to launch and fully implement this BPC-H effort and should help determine whether adjustments in the scope, scale, or timeline will be needed if the resources fall short.

Generic Metrics for Medical Training in Phase II

With an endorsed plan, broad consultation, some hedging options, and the requisite resources in place, the theater commands are ready to launch the BPC-H activity in the partner nation. Experts consulted for this study and previous research suggest that the effort should begin with a limited pilot program before full-scale implementation.[10] This may involve assessing the results of the initial medical-skill course to determine whether requirements for full-scale implementation have been met and identifying and modifying the program as needed. Metrics in this phase would assess whether the base plan is working correctly or whether hedging options need to be considered, thereby informing decisionmakers about readiness for full-scale implementation.

Metric 5: Adequacy of contact points and regular consultations. Communication is important to success. Knowing whom to contact for coordination, approvals, feedback, and assistance to clear bottlenecks is critical. Definitive contact points must be established within entities critical to implementation of activities. A measure for this metric might be frequency of communication with key persons and offices. Indicators could include a list of such key persons and offices, how to access them, and a schedule for regular consultation. Participation of

---

[10] See for example, Hartwig, Humphries, and Matebeni, 2008; Tang et al., 2005; Rowe et al., 2010; Moroney, Grissom, and Marquis, 2007.

these individuals and offices can help maintain interest in the effort and can support the subsequent train-the-trainer activities of the local military. Another indicator is the performance of conflict-resolution mechanisms to keep important audiences engaged and working cooperatively to achieve the desired outcomes of the BPC-H effort.

Metric 6: Level of success in recruiting trainees and conducting training. Capacity building is ultimately about expanding capabilities in persons, facilities, and institutions. Where training is concerned, the first step is to recruit the right trainees. If persons are not motivated to learn, they are not likely to be motivated to use their newly learned skills or transfer the skills to others.

One measure for success is recruitment. Indicators would be the number of recruited trainees vis-à-vis the target number of recruits and the number who meet entry requirements (e.g., skill sets that align with required skills, if any). Indicators for measuring success in training (both in knowledge and skills and as trainers) may be the performance of the recruits in tests and evaluations by trainers.

Metric 7: Level of partner performance. Since the local military will conduct training activities to extend new medical skills to a larger community of first responders and caregivers in the partner nation, it is important to understand the level of institutional capacity the local military has to conduct such activities.

Measures need to focus on assessing readiness and absorption capacity. Indicators should include the level of alignment between the partner nation's commitment of personnel and resources and the plan to carry out train-the-trainer activities on the targeted medical skills. At this point, the plan for sending local military trainers to the field—whether it is a joint U.S.-partner plan or an independent-partner plan—should be examined for critical assumptions and hedge options. This will enable the U.S. military to work with other supporters to assist the local military in harnessing the requirements to implement the train-the-trainer activities.

Metric 8: Readiness to scale up. Phase II is the opportunity for U.S. military organizations, the local military, and other stakeholders to test, learn, and make appropriate adjustments to the activity and to decide if the BPC-H effort is ready to move into full-scale implementation. Data from metrics 5, 6, and 7 (as well as assessment of resources, political will, etc.) will help to inform this decision.

An important indicator is the presence of resources necessary for full implementation. Also, lessons learned from Phase II need to documented. These lessons can help in the review and revision of assumptions in the plan and in making adjustments that may be necessary to scale up to full implementation. Lessons learned may pertain to critical communication with local elders, coordination with the health ministry, or internal accounting practices—anything that can affect the operation of processes in the BPC-H effort.

Generic Metrics for Medical Training in Phase III

With initial implementation confirmed as a success, the BPC-H effort moves into full-scale implementation. Metrics will continue to focus on collecting data on the performance of the process and partner capacity. Results of activities will also be documented. The number of local military personnel trained will be tallied, along with whether they have acquired knowledge and skills from the training and whether the local military is capable of conducting train-the-trainer activities on the new skills. If data and analysis indicate that the local military is not prepared for this task, the goal of increasing capacity in the public health sector will not have been achieved. This is also the time to begin assessing whether the BPC-H effort is creating corollary benefits for U.S. military organizations involved, e.g., deepening the experience of U.S. military personnel in cross-cultural communication and expanding awareness of local traditions, issues, and power brokers.

Metric 9: Effectiveness and Efficiency of Processes. At this stage, the GCC/TSOC, AFSOC, and other U.S. military health advisors continue to monitor performance of key processes, e.g., identifying the right local military personnel for training or assessing the effectiveness of medical-skill certification tests and the local ability to administer them.

Measures here focus on the effectiveness and efficiency of the processes described above. Indicators may include the number of local military personnel recruited for training versus the number completing the training,[11] along with their performance (low or high scores) on certification tests and trainer evaluations. U.S. health advisors and local military partners should both gain experience over time in teaching the course and selecting the right personnel to receive training. As such, the ratio between those who enter the course and those who pass it should improve with each subsequent class, and the performance of the trainees should also be expected to improve over time.

Indicators for the performance of consultation processes and conflict-resolution mechanisms are also important. As the BPC-H effort expands into full-scale implementation, new issues may emerge. Consultations with important audiences will be essential to help the local military succeed in reaching out to first-responder and caregiver communities to recruit trainees, help them integrate the new medical skills into their work, and persuade the communities they serve to accept the use of new techniques.

Metric 10: Results of immediate outputs and intermediate outcomes over time. The immediate output of this illustrative BPC-H program is clear, with the indicator being the number of local military medical personnel trained. With full-scale implementation of training, local medics who have completed their training should be going out into the field to treat citizens and train first responders and caregivers. Thus, the intermediate outcome would be the number of first responders and caregivers who received training from local military personnel and the number that met certification standards. Analysis of the data would show that (1) building capacity in the partner military has taken root (the local personnel are able to train others with minimal support from U.S. military health advisors), (2) the community of first responders and caregivers capable of using the new medical techniques is expanding, and (3) the target capacity of local trainers is being sustained over time.

At this point, it may not be clear whether an improvement in health outcomes (e.g., for emergency obstetrics, a drop in maternal mortality rates) can be observed or whether BPC-H efforts are having an effect on the local population's trust in local and national authorities or on its susceptibility to inroads by insurgent or terrorist groups.[12] Anecdotal evidence of improved ties between local military and communities that benefited from access to improved medical techniques or of cases of lives saved through the application of a new medical skill could at

---

[11] U.S. health-care advisors will need to continuously gauge whether the local military personnel can be trained. They cannot assume that everyone will be able to learn and perform satisfactorily. If there is a high noncompletion/fail rate, U.S. advisors will need to ascertain whether the personnel selected for training are appropriate. If not, interventions may be necessary to expand the number of recruits who will be more likely to complete/pass the course. Another option might be to look elsewhere for recruits, e.g., local hospitals, but that could be a hedge that would constitute a significant change in the BPC-H effort.

[12] One indicator might be an up-tick in information on extremist groups shared by community members with the local military, but it will be difficult to link this directly to the BPC-H effort.

least begin to indicate positive trends. Such evidence could also help inform the partner government and other supporters of the effort to look for ways to extend training opportunities and to expand acceptance of the new techniques in the indigenous society. In this sense, stories can be powerful tools. Documenting them and involving local partners, associates, and beneficiaries in retelling them can support communication to important stakeholders. It can also support outreach to communities that have yet to embrace the new medical techniques or the local government as an ally in development. Of course, as it accumulates, anecdotal evidence becomes data for more-rigorous analysis.

Metric 11. Impact on U.S. military training and access. BPC-H activities may expand training opportunities that help U.S. military personnel gain experience in cross-cultural environments. They may also expand advisors' access to elites in the local military and government. Since U.S. military health advisors would at this point be working most directly with the partner-nation military, it would be reasonable to begin assessing whether access and influence appear to be expanding. Whether U.S.-partner relations are positively affected and whether the local images of the partner and U.S. governments are improving may be better assessed later in the effort.

The indicators might include satisfaction ratings of U.S. military health advisors who trained local personnel and the level of communication and coordination between U.S. advisors and local counterparts. Measures would focus on whether the advisors conclude that the experience improved their readiness for deployment for this or similar types of missions and expanded their ability to work in cross-cultural settings. Another indicator would be assessments by personnel directly involved in training, planning, and other activities of whether the BPC-H effort had expanded their awareness of and access to individuals and organizations in the local military and government. The knowledge and insights gained, as well as the professional networks created, could be invaluable for the BPC-H effort and for the overall ability of U.S. advisors to engage with the partner nation.

Generic Metrics for Medical Training in Phase IV

In the final phase, if full-scale implementation has gone well and has met the expectations of key stakeholders, the partner is expected to take over the BPC-H effort. This means the local military and health ministry would be responsible for sustaining train-the-trainer activities, and the U.S. advisors would largely exit from the effort.

Metric 12: Readiness for hand-over. Data collected in Phase III on process effectiveness and efficiency, partner performance, and immediate outputs and intermediate outcomes are all useful for informing theater health-engagement planners whether the time is right to exit. If the Phase III monitoring indicates that processes do not work, the local military's performance is below par, and immediate outputs are scarce and intermediate outcomes nonexistent, the BPC-H effort would not appear ready to be handed over. In such a situation, a U.S. military exit could cause the effort to collapse, because there is no indication that the partner can sustain it or that any other entity can step in to do so. Moreover, exiting without any show of accomplishment could tarnish the U.S. military's reputation in the partner nation, along with that of the United States overall; undoing such damage can be costly, difficult, and time-consuming. If conditions prevent reasonable remedies from being attempted and suggest that U.S. advisors abandon the preferred option of a hand-over to local authorities, an orderly wrap-up of the effort that limits damage to relationships with local authorities and populations would be better than allowing the effort to conclude in chaos. Alternatively, theater health-engagement planners might seek an NGO to work with ministries in the partner government to continue training efforts with civilian providers.

On the other hand, if the metrics show high performance in processes to recruit and train local military medical personnel and expansion of partner capacity to acquire and transfer the new medical techniques, this suggests that the theater commands can proceed with hand-over and can begin withdrawing from the BPC-H effort.

If performance is satisfactory overall but there is some uncertainty about whether the time is right for the U.S. military to exit the effort, the theater commands should consider whether to extend involvement for another stretch of time until conditions for withdrawal are more promising. Additional indicators may be evidence of local government commitment to expanding training in and adoption of the targeted medical skills—e.g., in the form of new leadership, funding, and/or efforts to win the support of influential persons and organizations.

Metric 13: Level of benefit to the partner nation and the United States. At this point, an assessment might be made of how well the BPC-H effort has served mutual partner and U.S. interests and whether it has improved U.S. influence and access. The assessment could evaluate whether the program has increased indigenous capacity to train local first responders and caregivers in the new medical techniques; strengthened U.S.-partner military and diplomatic ties; improved the image of U.S. and partner military forces and governments; expanded training opportunities and cross-cultural work experience for AFSOC and other U.S. military health advisors; and enhanced U.S. awareness of conditions in high-risk areas in OEF-TS regions. One key indicator could be whether each side seeks opportunities for BPC-H efforts in other health-care sectors. Indicators of U.S. influence and access could measure levels of information-sharing and coordination between the United States and the partner.[13]

Identifying the right measures and indicators for improving the image of local military forces and governments as well as U.S. presence may be difficult. Impressions of beneficiaries, their families, and the communities that benefit from the new medical techniques may be biased and short-term. Also, if community-based first responders and caregivers deliver the targeted health-care techniques, it is not clear whether the government role would be evident to the beneficiaries, thereby affecting their impressions of local authorities. Nevertheless, acceptance of modern, Western health practices (potentially adapted to local cultural conditions) may at least be a short-term proxy indicator of a more positive image of the United States. Also, the willingness of local health-care workers to train under military personnel may be an indicator of a more positive local perception of the government and its institutions. Any greater willingness of communities in general to share information about local security and safety concerns with the military and other central government security forces may also be a proxy indicator of greater trust in the government. The benefit of increased awareness of conditions in high-risk areas would need to be assessed in terms of whether the information or insights gained would fill a critical gap or add value to U.S. medical and other intelligence.

Finally, BPC-H activities are aimed at improving health outcomes, and thus these outcomes must be tracked. It would be essential over the long term for relevant organizations such as NGOs to track, for example, the mortality rates of women who die or suffer serious health problems as a result of pregnancy and labor in communities that have adopted techniques for basic life-saving in obstetrics. In the short and medium term, more-appropriate measures and

---

[13] See Haims et al., 2011, Table 3.2, p. 33.

indicators may be the number of communities receiving training from local military personnel, whether new techniques have gained widespread acceptance and use, and whether the number of local communities requesting training in new medical skills from local military or other government personnel is increasing.

Conclusion

The framework introduced in this chapter can help conceptualize a phased approach to a BPC-H effort. The generic metrics and supporting measures and indicators for health engagement in less-developed countries presented here provide a construct for needed data-gathering and analysis to inform theater commands and other stakeholders about the management of a BPC-H effort and to demonstrate progress, challenges, and achievements. Metrics are tools, and having the right metrics and supporting measures and indicators can help monitor performance, motivate participants to work toward achieving shared objectives, and assess effectiveness. The construct described here provides a guide for developing, implementing, and assessing a BPC-H program; greater specificity on timelines, project phases, and metrics will be required for particular projects in selected partner nations.

The generic metrics and associated measures and indicators described in this chapter and the conceptual framework toward which they would be applied were designed to provide a comprehensive perspective in assessing the effectiveness of BPC-H activities. Ultimately, it will be necessary to select the right metrics and supporting measures and indicators to inform the theater commands of the most important things to monitor to assess the performance and effectiveness of a BPC-H effort.

CHAPTER FIVE

Findings and Recommendations

The study described in this report seeks to place health security in the context of U.S. strategy and U.S. efforts to build partner capacity and to recommend ways of maximizing the effectiveness of what we term BPC-H—building partner health capacity involving U.S. military forces. In light of the increasing emphasis in DoD on influencing "relevant populations," new direction on medical stability operations, and AFSOC's concept, RAND researchers examined the status of health engagement as a requirement in DoD guidance and military strategy and AFSOC's role in planning for and conducting BPC-H missions in support of USSOCOM and GCC objectives. They also analyzed organizations that have pursued activities that are similar to or otherwise relevant to BPC-H efforts in order to gain insights into successful practices that the GCCs, TSOCs, and components such as AFSOC might apply to their own efforts. Finally, they developed a framework for assessing and tracking health engagement efforts.

This chapter summarizes the study's key findings and provides a set of recommendations for USAF in general and AFSOC in particular on ways to maximize the effectiveness of efforts to build partner health capacity. The recommendations should also be of interest to GCCs and TSOCs.

Key Findings

Theater commands are the key to closing the gap between guidance and execution of BPC-H efforts. DoD recognizes that defeating extremist threats requires influencing relevant populations and that helping partners extend governance to those populations, particularly by providing health care, is critical to enhancing well-being and improving the legitimacy of local authorities in the eyes of their citizens. There is ample guidance that sets forth an operational requirement to build partner health capacity. DoDI 6000.16 directs the military health system to organize, train, and equip forces for medical stability operations. However, few U.S. military health operations overseas have executed this mission in a systematic and sustained manner. With recent guidance, theater commands are directed to put emphasis on medical stability operations in their plans, and these commands need to direct and source them. BPC-H missions are relatively inexpensive, but their return can be substantial in terms of both supporting partners and avoiding the need for and cost of later intervention.

Efforts to build partner health capacity can be either supported or supporting operations. DoDI 6000.16 further affords medical operations a priority comparable to that of combat operations. Although traditionally viewed by commanders as *supporting* operations, activities to build partner health capacity can be *supported* operations in some circumstances.

Conditions may exist in some regions or countries that preclude the U.S. military from training, advising, and assisting existing or potential partners in kinetic capabilities, but health engagement can help "get a foot in the door" and may be a primary means of gaining access and initiating relationships.

The U.S. Air Force can play an important role in building partner military health capacity. USAF considers building partnerships and partner capacity as one of its core functions, and its medical personnel are tasked to support GCC theater-engagement strategies around the world. USAF serves as executive agent for DIMO and provides training teams for disaster preparedness to foreign countries. Moreover, USAF's IHSs, competent not only in medical skills but also in foreign languages and regional knowledge, provide a unique capability to MAJCOMs and GCC commanders. Thus, USAF is well positioned to expand its role in health engagement.

AFSOC's BPC-H "niche" in the near term appears to be the mission itself. Very few military organizations are systematically pursuing BPC-H as defined here, yet the demand is great. As long as AFSOC health advisors serve as "go-to" professionals for the BPC-H mission, AFSOC's niche is the mission itself. However, as USAF meets guidance by organizing, equipping, and training its medical personnel to conduct systematic BPC-H activities, AFSOC health advisors will need to define a more specific niche for their capabilities within the mission. It is therefore important for medical planners to account for ongoing nonmilitary health capacity-building efforts in potential partner countries and to identify "best-fit" opportunities.

Successfully building and sustaining partner health capacity in less-developed regions requires long-term effort and commitment in synchronization with other military and civilian agencies and organizations, and this may conflict with shorter-term theater-command priorities. Without long-term, focused support for BPC-H missions from DoD and the GCCs and TSOCs, health engagement will be sporadic and may not make the impact that it could make. Such support will be key to the success of BPC-H, because control of taskings to health advisors rests with these commands. Assignment of an AFSOC medical planner to the SOCAFRICA staff can help the TSOC understand AFSOC's specific capabilities and can help AFSOC get involved with the TSOC's BPC-H planning.

Given the previous finding and the need to involve multiple stakeholders in BPC-H programs, well-defined, multiyear plans are critical to success. From the outset, plans for enhancing a partner's capacity in a specific health-care sector must be realistic and based on careful, in-depth assessment of the environment in which the BPC-H effort will take place. In addition, plans must be flexible enough to adjust for contingencies such as failure to meet benchmarks, altered participation of associated organizations, and crises that render BPC-H–tasked health advisors unavailable for periods of time.

Recommendations for AFSOC

Communicate the BPC-H concept and approach to external audiences frequently. Direction and resources for the BPC-H mission will require buy-in from USAF (the Surgeon General of the Air Force has already expressed support for the AFSOC concept), DoD, the theater commands, the interagency community, and the wider development community. It will be essential for AFSOC health advisors to communicate the AFSOC concept in order to generate greater appreciation among key stakeholders for the contribution that BPC-H can make to both U.S. and partner interests. AFSOC advisors can also learn a great deal through such interactions. AFSOC should leverage public affairs opportunities to explain BPC-H efforts whenever possible.

In developing plans with theater commands for BPC-H programs, consider scheduling multiple visits per year and throughout the duration of U.S. military involvement. Visits should be driven not only by the needs of the plan, but also by the high-value relationships that can be built with partner nations over time. "One-off" visits—those for which there is little or no follow-up—do not usually build and sustain partner capacity, especially in less-developed nations. In fact, they can harm relationships by raising expectations that are not fulfilled.

Engage stakeholders early in the planning process and in program development and design. Building partner military capacity in health is often undertaken in the context of efforts by civilian organizations (such as USAID) to work with partner health ministries and civilian medical communities. Among the first stakeholders AFSOC and the supported GCC/TSOC must engage are the U.S. embassy team in the target country and the partner government itself. The latter may include not only the military, but also the ministries of health, agriculture, and finance and other relevant civilian agencies. Importantly, potential associates such as NGOs should be included in the planning process, as they need time to plan and execute their participation in a program.

Assess the effectiveness of BPC-H activities according to both military and developmental measures. The four-phase conceptual approach to planning for, implementing, and assessing the effectiveness of health engagement developed in this study is based on an understanding of both developmental and military requirements. The suggested metrics should help monitor alignment of implementation with goals and plans in both realms. AFSOC and the theater commands will need to show success based on both developmental and military metrics to continue generating support for the BPC-H mission among existing and potential stakeholders.

Approach early BPC-H excursions with an eye toward learning lessons and adapting procedures based on experience. Engagement in OEF-TS countries offers an opportunity for USAFRICOM, SOCAFRICA, and AFSOC to critically examine the approach to health engagement. Advisors may need to collect additional data about the effort itself to learn from and assess the challenges faced in early efforts. Thus, theater and AFSOC planners might consider two mission reports—one containing metrics on the impact of interactions with the partner nation and other stakeholders and one that assesses the process of planning and executing BPC-H—with the understanding that each case may present unique challenges.

Consider the "risk" of success. This recommendation may seem counterintuitive, but success breeds demand. The more AFSOC and other U.S. military organizations demonstrate their ability to help less-developed partners extend governance, improve the well-being of relevant populations, and reduce vulnerability to extremism, the greater the demand will be for health advisors. Given other critical taskings, including force health protection and casualty care, AFSOC will need to assist tasking commands in evaluating the trade-offs they are implicitly making between BPC-H and other taskings.

Recommendations for USAF

Examine whether and how AFSOC's BPC-H concept and approach are scalable to the general-purpose Air Force. It is not clear whether AFSOC's approach to planning and executing health engagement can be scaled up to the wider Air Force or used in other USAF MAJCOMs. If USAF is to embrace the BPC-H mission in a systematic fashion, it will need to examine AFSOC's approach and determine how it can be applied on a larger scale.

Consider dedicating some USAF- and/or MAJCOM-level resources to forming a cadre of medical personnel with regional focus and expertise in BPC-H planning and execution. The IHS program is the only one of its kind in the U.S. military, and it has demonstrated its utility. But it is small, and IHS professionals have a relatively broad charter as members of GCC staffs and MAJCOMs. The Air Force might determine whether a BPC-H–dedicated cadre (potentially including an expanded IHS program) is warranted. Resources required to form such a cadre are likely to be minimal if organizational alignments (i.e., in the Air Staff and the MAJCOMs) and training for selected personnel in the Air Force Medical Service can be adjusted. In particular, training should include cross-cultural communication, language, and medical planning and execution for efforts in nations that have inadequate, dissimilar health systems and infrastructures.

Concluding Remarks

The U.S. military has an important role to play in building the health-care capacity of governments in less-developed nations. Working with partner militaries and with other U.S., partner-nation, and international organizations, the U.S. military can help improve the capacity of local authorities to deliver services to their most vulnerable citizens, enhance the legitimacy of these authorities in the eyes of the communities they serve, and—it is hoped—prevent violent extremist groups from taking root in and exploiting undergoverned territories. Health-care capacity-building activities can be planned and implemented in pursuit of both developmental and military objectives.

The need to conduct BPC-H efforts systematically and in a sustained way suggests that the processes within the military for planning and executing these activities also need to be systematic and sustained. The Services and the combatant commands will need to provide resources not only for BPC-H operations in the field, but also for capable medical planners on planning staffs and a training pipeline to sustain a BPC-H cadre. Policies, processes, and systems will need to be developed and implemented to ensure that BPC-H can be carried out effectively. A crucial next step is to delineate the portion of the demand for BPC-H that is appropriate for the U.S. military to address, and then to determine how this demand can be addressed through resource allocation and systems redesign.

Bibliography

12th Air Force, "Medical Readiness Training Exercises (MEDRETEs)," Fact Sheet, June 24, 2008. As of March 8, 2012:
http://www.12af.acc.af.mil/library/factsheets/factsheet.asp?id=7694

"95th CA BDE Personnel Excel File," U.S. Army Force Management Support Agency (USAFMSA), website, undated.

"95th CA BDE Command Slide Brief," Fort Bragg, NC, March 10, 2010.

AFSOC—*See* Air Force Special Operations Command.

Air Force Special Operations Command, "6th Special Operations Squadron: Combat Aviation Advisors," briefing, Hurlburt Air Force Base, Fla., April 2006.

———, "AFSOC Combat Aviation Advisor Mission Qualification Course," March 27, 2009a.

———, "AFSOC Medical Support for Irregular Warfare (IW), Healthcare Engagement (HE), Stability, Security, Transition and Reconstruction (SSTR) Operations," background paper, October 2009b.

Alderman, Maj Shawn, et al., "Medical Seminars: A New Paradigm for SOF COIN Medical Programs," *Journal of Special Operations Medicine*, Vol. 10, Ed. 1, Winter 2010, pp. 16–22.

Army Training Requirements and Resources System, website, 2010. As of July 10, 2010:
https://www.atrrs.army.mil

Baker, Jay B., "Medical Diplomacy in Full-Spectrum Operations," *Military Review*, September–October 2007, pp. 63–73.

Bhargava, Vinay Kumar, *Global Issues for Global Citizens*, Washington, D.C.: The World Bank Group, 2006, pp. 341–370.

Bricknell, M., and D. Thompson, "Roles for International Military Medical Services in Stability Operations (Security Sector Reform)," *Journal of Royal Army Medical Corps*, Vol. 153, No. 2, September 2007, pp. 95–98.

Brown, Lisanne, Anne LaFond, and Kate McIntyre, *Measuring Capacity Building*, Chapel Hill, N.C.: University of North Carolina at Chapel Hill, March 2001. As of October 21, 2010:
http://www.heart-intl.net/HEART/Financial/comp/MeasuringCapacityBuilg.pdf

Cahill, Capt Mike, "Lessons Learned from Cooperative Medical Engagements 08–09," 172nd Battalion Surgeon, U.S. Army, briefing, April 28, 2009.

Cariappa, M. P., B. K. Mohanti, and E. V. Bonventre, "Operation Sadbhavana: Winning Hearts and Minds in the Ladakh Himalayan Region," *Military Medicine*, Vol. 173, No. 8, August 2008, pp. 749–753.

Cecchine, Gary, and Melinda Moore, *Infectious Disease and National Security: Strategic Information Needs*, Santa Monica, Calif.: RAND Corporation, TR-405-OSD, 2006. As of March 8, 2012:
http://www.rand.org/pubs/technical_reports/TR405.html

Center for Reproductive Rights, "Rights Group Targets Maternal Deaths in Mali," February 4, 2002. As of March 8, 2012:
http://reproductiverights.org/en/press-room/rights-groups-target-maternal-death-in-mali

Craddock, General Bantz J., Commander, U.S. European Command, Statement Before the House Armed Services Committee, March 13, 2008.

Dewar, James A., Carl H. Builder, William M. Hix, and Morlie Levin, *Assumption-Based Planning: A Planning Tool for Very Uncertain Times*, Santa Monica, Calif.: RAND Corporation, MR-114-A, 1993. As of March 8, 2012:
http://www.rand.org/pubs/monograph_reports/MR114.html

DIMO, "Defense Institute for Medical Operations: Course Catalog," USAFSAM/ETE, Brooks Air Force Base, Texas, undated.

Dixon, Thomas Homer, *The Ingenuity Gap*, New York, NY: Random House, 2000.

Foreign Policy, "The Failed States Index 2009," website, 2009. As of March 8, 2012:
http://www.foreignpolicy.com/articles/2009/06/22/the_2009_failed_states_index

———, "The Failed States Index 2010," website, 2010. As of December 6, 2010:
http://www.foreignpolicy.com/articles/2010/06/21/2010_failed_states_index_interactive_map_and_rankings

Gates, Robert M., "Helping Others Defend Themselves: The Future of U.S. Security Assistance," *Foreign Affairs*, Vol. 89, No. 3, May/June 2010.

Grub, Michael, "6 SOS Combat Aviation Advisors," Air Force Special Operations Command, Hurlburt Field, Fla., briefing, May 2010.

Haims, Marla C., Melinda Moore, Harold D. Green, Jr., and Cynthia Clapp-Wincek, *Developing a Prototype Handbook for Monitoring and Evaluating Department of Defense Humanitarian Assistance Projects*, Santa Monica, Calif.: RAND Corporation, TR-784-OSD, 2011. As of March 8, 2012:
http://www.rand.org/pubs/technical_reports/TR784.html

Hale, Joseph V., "Medical Diplomacy: A Critique of the U.S. Air Force Model," Air Command College, Air University, thesis, 2008.

Hartwig, Kari A., Debbie Humphries, and Zethu Matebeni, "Building Capacity for AIDS NGOs in Southern Africa: Evaluation of a Pilot Initiative," *Health Promotion International*, Vol. 23, No. 3, April 2008.

Hauser, John R., and Gerald M. Katz, "Metrics: You Are What You Measure!" April 1998. As of October 21, 2010:
http://www.mit.edu/~hauser/Papers/Hauser-Katz%20Measure%2004-98.pdf

Health Affairs, "About the Journal," webpage, 2010. As of December 13, 2010:
http://www.healthaffairs.org/1500_about_journal.php

Huynh, Mylene T., "Air Force Medical Service Building Partnership Capabilities," briefing, AFMSA/XGSI, Arlington, Va., May 27, 2010.

Iddins, Brig Gen Bart O., "Irregular Warfare Healthcare Engagement," AFSOC, undated.

"Joint Task Force-Haiti Mission Update Brief," provided by 95th CA BDE staff officers, February 12, 2010.

Jones, Seth G., Lee H. Hilborne, C. Ross Anthony, Lois M. Davis, Federico Girosi, Cheryl Benard, Rachel M. Swanger, Anita Datar Garten and Anga R. Timilsina, *Securing Health: Lessons from Nation-Building Missions*, Santa Monica, Calif.: RAND Corporation, MG-321-RC, 2006. As of March 8, 2012:
http://www.rand.org/pubs/monographs/MG321.html

Kirby, Julia, "Towards a Theory of High Performance" *Harvard Business Review*, July/August 2005, pp. 30–39.

Krueger, Mary V., "Medical Diplomacy in the United States Army: A Concept Whose Time Has Come," Fort Leavenworth, Kan.: U.S. Army Command and General Staff College, thesis, 2008. As of March 8, 2012:
http://www.dtic.mil/cgi-bin/GetTRDoc?Location=U2&doc=GetTRDoc.pdf&AD=ADA483047

Lambooy, J. G., "Knowledge Transfers, Spillovers and Actors: The Role of Context and Social Capital," *European Planning Studies*, Vol. 18, No. 6, June 2010, pp. 873–891.

Lightsey, Ross F., Sr., "Persistent Engagement: Civil Military Support Elements Operating in CENTCOM," *Special Warfare*, Vol. 23, Issue 3, May/June 2010.

Malsby, Robert Franklin III, "Into Which End Does the Thermometer Go? Application of Military Medicine in Counterinsurgency: Does Direct Patient Care by American Service Members Work?" Fort Leavenworth, Kan.: U.S. Army Command and General Staff College, thesis, 2008. As of March 8, 2012:
http://fhpr.osd.mil/intlhealth/pdfs/Thesis(Final)forprint.pdf

Marquis, Jefferson P., Jennifer D. P. Moroney, Justin Beck, Derek Eaton, Scott Hiromoto, David R. Howell, Janet Lewis, Charlotte Lynch, Michael J. Neumann, and Cathryn Quantic Thurston, *Developing an Army Strategy for Building Partner Capacity for Stability Operations*, Santa Monica, Calif.: RAND Corporation, MG-942-A, 2010. As of March 8, 2012:
http://www.rand.org/pubs/monographs/MG942.html

McCawley, Paul F., "The Logic Model for Program Planning and Evaluation," University of Idaho Extension, CIS 1097, 1997. As of October 21, 2010:
http://www.uiweb.uidaho.edu/extension/LogicModel.pdf

Moroney, Jennifer D. P., Kim Cragin, Eric Stephen Gons, Beth Grill, John E. Peters, and Rachel M. Swanger, *International Cooperation with Partner Air Forces*, Santa Monica, Calif.: RAND Corporation, MG-790-AF, 2009. As of March 8, 2012:
http://www.rand.org/pubs/monographs/MG790.html

Moroney, Jennifer D. P., Adam Grissom, and Jefferson P. Marquis, *A Capabilities-Based Strategy for Army Security Cooperation*, Santa Monica, Calif.: RAND Corporation, MG-563-A, 2007. As of March 8, 2012:
http://www.rand.org/pubs/monographs/MG563.html

Moroney, Jennifer D. P., Joe Hogler, Jefferson P. Marquis, Christopher Paul, John E. Peters, and Beth Grill, *Developing an Assessment Framework for U.S. Air Force Building Partnerships Programs*, Santa Monica, Calif.: RAND Corporation, MG-868-AF, 2010. As of March 8, 2012:
http://www.rand.org/pubs/monographs/MG868.html

National Intelligence Council, *Global Trends 2015: A Dialogue About the Future with Nongovernment Experts*, Washington, D.C., December 2000.

National Partnership for Reinventing Government, "Balancing Measures: Best Practice in Performance Management," August 1999. As of December 14, 2010:
http://govinfo.library.unt.edu/npr/library/papers/bkgrd/balmeasure.html

Olson, Admiral Eric T., *Statement Before the Senate Armed Services Committee on the Posture of Special Operations Forces,* March 2009.

Parr, Sakiko Fukuda, Carlos Lopes, Kalid Malik, and Mark Mallock Braun, eds., *Capacity for Development: New Solutions to Old Problems*, London: Earthscan Books/UNDP, 2002.

Petit, Brian, "OEF-Philippines: Thinking COIN, Practicing FID," *Special Warfare*, Vol. 23, No. 1, January–February 2010, pp. 10–15.

Project HOPE, "About Us," webpage, undated. As of March 8, 2012:
http://www.projecthope.org/about/

———, "Financial Information," webpage, undated. As of December 13, 2010:
http://www.projecthope.org/site/PageServer?pagename=about_us_financials

———, "Where We Work," webpage, undated. As of December 14, 2010:
http://www.projecthope.org/where-we-work/

———, 2009 Annual Report: A Community of HOPE, Millwood, Va., 2009. As of March 8, 2012:
http://donate.projecthope.org/site/DocServer/HPE_AR09-spreads.pdf?docID=261

Rice, Susan E., and Stewart Patrick, "Index of State Weakness in the Developing World," The Brookings Institution, 2008. As of March 8, 2012:
http://www.brookings.edu/reports/2008/02_weak_states_index.aspx

Rowe, Laura A., Sister B. Brillant, et al., "Building Capacity in Health Facilities Management: Guiding Principles for Skills Transfer in Liberia," *Human Resources for Health*, Vol. 8, No. 5, 2010.

"Special Operations Forces: Training with Friendly Foreign Forces," Title 10 of the U.S. Code, Section 2011. As of March 8, 2012:
http://codes.lp.findlaw.com/uscode/10/A/III/101/2011

Sun, Peter Y. T., and H. A. Marc, "An Examination of the Relationship Between Absorptive Capacity and Organizational Learning and a Proposed Integration," *International Journal of Management Reviews*, Vol. 12, No. 2, November 27, 2008, pp. 130–150.

Tang, Kwok-Cho, Don Nutbeam, et al., "Building Capacity for Health Promotion—A Case Study of China," *Health Promotion International*, Vol. 20, No. 3, March 2005.

Thaler, David E., *Strategies to Tasks: A Framework for Linking Means and Ends*, Santa Monica, Calif.: RAND Corporation, MR-300-AF, 1993. As of March 8, 2012:
http://www.rand.org/pubs/monograph_reports/MR300.html

Transparency International, "Corruption Perceptions Index 2009," website, undated. As of March 8, 2012:
http://www.transparency.org/policy_research/surveys_indices/cpi/2009/cpi_2009_table

———, "Corruption Perceptions Index 2010 Results," website, undated. As of December 6,2010: http://www.transparency.org/policy_research/surveys_indices/cpi/2010/results

United Nations Development Program, "Human Development Index (HDI)—2010 Rankings," Human Development Reports webpage, undated. As of December 6, 2010:
http://hdr.undp.org/en/statistics/

USACAPOC, "Civil Affairs General Officer Steering Committee Slides," Fort Bragg, NC, April 27, 2010.

U.S. Africa Command, "Operation Enduring Freedom Trans Sahara," website, undated. As of November 29, 2010:
http://www.africom.mil/oef-ts.asp

U.S. Agency for International Development, Health, "Countries," web site, undated. As of March 8, 2012:
http://www.usaid.gov/our_work/global_health/home/Countries/

———, Office of U.S. Foreign Disaster Assistance (OFDA), "Haiti—Earthquake," Fact Sheet #55, Fiscal Year (FY) 2010, May 21, 2010a. As of August 2010:
http://www.usaid.gov/our_work/humanitarian_assistance/disaster_assistance/countries/haiti/template/fs_sr/fy2010/haiti_eq_fs55_05-21-2010.pdf

———, Office of U.S. Foreign Disaster Assistance (OFDA), "Pakistan—Complex Emergency and Landslide," Fact Sheet #10, Fiscal Year (FY) 2010, July 15, 2010b. As of March 8, 2012:
http://www.usaid.gov/our_work/humanitarian_assistance/disaster_assistance/countries/pakistan/template/fs_sr/fy2010/pakistan_ce_fs10_09-30-2010.pdf

U.S. Air Force, *Air Force Global Partnership Strategy: Building Partnerships for the 21st Century*, December 18, 2008.

———, *Enduring Airpower Lessons from OEF/OIF: Air Force Special Operations Command Aviation Foreign Internal Defense*, Office of Air Force Lessons Learned, August 24, 2009.

———, "6th Special Operations Squadron," Fact Sheet, website, 2010. As of December 6, 2010: http://www2.hurlburt.af.mil/library/factsheets/factsheet.asp?id=3496

U.S. Army, *Operations, Field Manual 3-0*, February 12, 2008.

———, *Civil Affairs Operations, Field Manual 3-57*, October 2011.

U.S. Department of Defense, "Military Support for Stability, Security, Transition, and Reconstruction (SSTR) Operations," DoD Directive 3000.05, November 28, 2005.

———, *Guidance for the Employment of the Force*, 2008a (not releasable to the general public).

———, *Irregular Warfare (IW)*, Washington, D.C.: Office of the Under Secretary of Defense for Policy, DoDD 3000.07, December 1, 2008b.

———, *National Defense Strategy*, June 2008c.

———, *Functional Needs Analysis for Stability Operations: Military Health System*, January 23, 2009.

———, *Quadrennial Defense Review Report*, February 2010a.

———, *DoD Dictionary of Military and Associated Terms*, Joint Publication 1-02, April 12, 2001 (as amended through April 2010b).

———, *Irregular Warfare: Countering Irregular Threats, Joint Operating Concept*, Version 2.0, May 2010c.

————, "Military Health Support for Stability Operations," DoD Instruction 6000.16, May 17, 2010d.

————, *Sustaining U.S. Global Leadership: Sustaining 21ˢᵗ Century Defense*, January 2012.

U.S. Government Accountability Office, , "Reports on the Government Performance and Results Act," website, undated. As of October 21, 2010:
http://www.gao.gov/new.items/gpra/gpra.htm

————, "Performance Measurement and Evaluation: Definitions and Relationships," May 2005.

U.S. Special Operations Command, "Priorities of USSOCOM," command website, 2010 (not accessible by the general public).

Vick, Alan J., Adam Grissom, William Rosenau, Beth Grill, and Karl P. Mueller, *Air Power in the New Counterinsurgency Era: The Strategic Importance of USAF Advisory and Assistance Missions*, Santa Monica, Calif.: RAND Corporation, MG-509-AF, 2006. As of March 8, 2012:
http://www.rand.org/pubs/monographs/MG509.html

Ward, William E., *Statement Before the Senate Armed Service Committee and House Armed Services Committee on the Posture of U.S. Africa Command*, March 10, 2010.

Wilder, Andrew, testimony presented at Hearing on U.S. Aid to Pakistan: Planning and Accountability, House Committee on Oversight and Government Reform, Subcommittee on National Security and Foreign Affairs, December 9, 2009.

Wilson, Gregory, "Anatomy of a Successful COIN Operation: OEF-Philippines and the Indirect Approach," *Military Review*, November–December 2006.

World Health Organization, "Mali Mortality Country Fact Sheet 2006," WHO Statistical Information System, Mortality Profiles, 2006. As of March 8, 2012:
www.afro.who.int/index.php?option=com_docman&task=doc_download&gid=1290